'*Invisibly Blighted* touches a nerve with a shar[...] society from the point of view of a child. How [...] How does childhood fit within a highly techn[...] parents respect the digital privacy of their child[...] with sexting? The authors reflect on these issues with their wit and heart, defining what it means to be human in a digital world.'

Dr Kari Kivinen, Head of the Lycée franco-finlandais d'Helsinki and former Secretary-General of the European Schools

'The way any society prepares and cares for its children is one of its toughest tests. In the twenty-first century, ideas about childhood, about what it means to be a child, are shifting as a result of rapid social, demographic and technological change. This book asks profound questions about how we discharge our responsibilities to children, and how we prepare them as the citizens of the future.'

Professor Chris Husbands, Vice-Chancellor, Sheffield Hallam University

'This book has the rare combination of plain language and real-world examples that can bring up to speed those of us interested in the impact of digital technology on childhood without making us feel old or out-of-date. It also doesn't shy away from difficult issues, meaning the read isn't always comfortable, but it's always fascinating.'

Laura McInerney, Editor, *Schools Week*

'This book is a timely examination of the new challenges facing children in a digital world. Parents, teachers and policymakers are all struggling to keep up with reality and would do well to read and debate what is covered here. As a legislator, I am grateful for the insights leading me to want a more sustainable balance between education and prohibition if we are to better support children.'

Lord Knight, Minister for Work and Pensions, 2009–10

'The authors offer a rare insight into the nuances of young people's lives online by talking with them rather than at them. Without an understanding of children's experience, those who are tasked with ensuring their safety are doomed to fail.'

Wendy M. Grossman, Author, journalist, and blogger

'The overlap between childhood and new digital playgrounds – and the challenges therein – is one of the most important new spaces for us to clarify, analyse and map, and Sandra Leaton Gray is one of our most readable, informed and convincing navigators. This book contributes enormously to our understanding of the perils, opportunities and implications that face our children and their adult counterparts.'

Tom Bennett, founder of researchED, author, and behaviour adviser to the Department for Education

Invisibly Blighted

It was as if, at moments, we were perpetually coming into sight of subjects before which we must stop short, turning suddenly out of alleys that we perceived to be blind, closing with a little bang that made us look at each other – for, like all bangs, it was something louder than we had intended – the doors we had indiscreetly opened.

Henry James, *The Turn of the Screw*

Invisibly Blighted

The digital erosion of childhood

Sandra Leaton Gray and
Andy Phippen

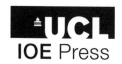
IOE Press

First published in 2017 by the UCL Institute of Education Press, University College London, 20 Bedford Way, London WC1H 0AL

www.ucl-ioe-press.com

British Library Cataloguing in Publication Data:
A catalogue record for this publication is available from the British Library

ISBNs
978-1-78277-050-3 (paperback)
978-1-78277-198-2 (PDF eBook)
978-1-78277-199-9 (ePub eBook)
978-1-78277-200-2 (Kindle eBook)

Typeset by Quadrant Infotech (India) Pvt Ltd
Printed by CPI Group (UK) Ltd, Croydon, CR0 4YY
Cover: *Kindlifresserbrunnen* (the Ogre Fountain, 1542–6) by Hans Gieng, in the Kornhausplatz, Bern. Photo by Andrew Bossi, reproduced under Creative Commons licence CC-BY-SA-2.5.

Contents

List of figures and tables

Acknowledgements

This book has been a long time in the writing, but as the journey progressed it seemed to become increasingly topical. We would like to thank the following people, who offered vital encouragement along the way.

Jim Collins and Nicky Platt from the UCL IOE Press for their patience with this project, UCL IOE colleagues Michael Reiss, Clare Brooks, Shirley Dex, and David Scott, former Cambridge colleague John McBeath, Plymouth colleague Megan Crawford, fellow members of the Privacy and Policy Expert Group of the Biometrics Institute (especially Isabelle Moeller, Ted Dunstone, Juliet Lodge, and Terry Aulich), Emmeline Taylor, Terri Dowty, Ross Anderson, and Pippa King. We are also indebted to David Speigelhalter and David Alexander for encouraging us to embark upon the study of risk in relation to childhood. We must also acknowledge the South West Grid for Learning Trust for their generosity with the 360 Degree Safe data, in particular David Wright and Ron Richards. We would like to thank the staff members who helped make the empirical work possible: Sue Hargreaves, Chris McDonald, Peter Binding, Sue Hodges, and Davina Bray. Finally, we must not forget all the children and young people that gave freely of their time and opinions when answering our questions, and we hope this book represents their views and concerns faithfully.

About the authors

Sandra Leaton Gray is Senior Lecturer in Education at the UCL Institute of Education. She is a former teacher and specialist in sociology of education, with a special interest in issues surrounding contemporary identity and technology. Sandra is also a member of the Privacy Expert Group of the Biometrics Institute, and a senior member of Wolfson College, Cambridge University. Sandra is the author of the book *Teachers Under Siege* (Trentham, 2006) and many articles and book chapters on the sociology of education, professionalism, biometrics, technology and identity. She appears regularly on radio and TV discussing childhood and schooling, and was featured in Lord Puttnam's documentary film on education *We Are The People We've Been Waiting For* (2009).

Andy Phippen is Professor of Children and Technology at the Plymouth University Business School. He has worked in a consultative capacity for more than twenty years with companies such as British Telecom, Google, and Facebook on issues of ethical and social responsibility. He has specialized in the use of ICT by children and young people for more than ten years, carrying out a large amount of grass roots research on issues such as their attitudes towards privacy and data protection, internet safety, and contemporary issues such as sexting and peer abuse. He has presented written and oral evidence to parliamentary enquiries related to children's use of ICT and is widely published in the area. He is a research partner with the UK Safer Internet Centre and is a frequent media commentator on children and the internet.

Chapter 1

What is childhood?

In the old centre of Berne, visitors to the Kornhausplatz are greeted with a very strange sight in the form of the sixteenth-century *Kindlifresserbrunnen* statue (Bernese German for 'child eating fountain'). This is a bizarre landmark consisting of a man apparently eating infant children. Its meaning and historical significance has been lost over the centuries, and continues to be debated, especially amongst the Swiss children it has presumably terrified for 500 years. For the purposes of this book, this somewhat alarming statue provides a useful image as we consider the confused and often ambivalent relationships between childhood, identity, and technology in the modern age. Such relationships are fraught with questions. As our children navigate a complex and highly connected social world fuelled by technology, how far are we helping them to grow into the adults we would wish them to be? Or are we in fact allowing their childhoods to be 'eaten' as we seek to develop and change society in the information age? What are the long term implications of this? To answer such questions, we start with the issue of childhood itself, along with the different philosophies and definitions that have been associated with it over recent centuries.

Conceptualizing childhood

How we conceptualize childhood depends on many things, not least our own stage of development and position within society. For example, when we were first commissioned to write this book, Sandra's youngest son Felix was four years old, which was a difficult concept for him and a fascinating one for her. On the one hand, Felix knew he was not a baby any longer. This was clear to him, as babies were associated with nappies, bottles, and pushchairs. He wanted to be certain he had left babyhood behind him, as he had worked out that there were many things babies couldn't do, such as walking, talking, and acting out Star Wars games with his elder brothers. That, for him, represented a significant deficit. He liked to think that he was bigger and better than that, and had moved on. On the other hand, however, Felix realized at four that he was not a proper big boy either. Big boys can read, play computer games involving text-based instructions, and count pocket money out by themselves. This leads to a degree of consumer freedom he could only aspire to at that time. Big boys go to big school, a mysterious place accessed by bus or train and involving wearing watches, blazers, and ties, something he associated with sophistication and scholarly progress. Even more exciting, big boys can reach into high kitchen cupboards to raid the biscuits, go on more exciting fairground rides than their little brothers, and talk to grown-ups without getting a crick in the neck. In the light of all of these things, Felix posed himself this question regularly: was he little, was he big, or was he both at the same time?

Of course, what Felix didn't realize was that his existential dilemma was something being played out every day, in every family's household across the land. The way we define notions of childhood can be very similar to Felix's categorizations at the tender age of four. There are biological deficits associated with youth, for example, such as being physically shorter or weaker than the majority of the population. There are cognitive deficits, such as not being able to read, tell the time, or count money properly. In addition there are social deficits, such as being expected to stay within a fairly limited geographical boundary, constantly supervised by adults, even if you can't see them watching you. Children are also perceived at different times as consumers (of goods and consumer products); chattels (in terms of being the property and responsibility of their parents); proto-adults (in terms of their dress); proto-delinquents (in terms of some members of society feeling threatened by them); and innocents (in terms of needing protection from the external environment). This is not happening in isolation. In all these different forms of twenty-first-century children's social identity, we see philosophical debates from history being played out on the contemporary stage. Considering these categorizations and the way they locate children within society is a good starting point for understanding childhood in the technological age.

Defining childhood

The very word 'childhood' is increasingly open to interpretation once attempts are made to define it more precisely. Over the last century or so, methods of defining childhood have proliferated and at the same time become more complex and confused (James and Prout, 2004; Palmer, 2006; Postman, 1994). In the midst of this, UNESCO's International Year of the Child in 1979 was a landmark attempt to take an overview and draw attention to the problems experienced by children throughout the world. A development of the Declaration of the Rights of the Child (1924/59), the International Year of the Child triggered a great deal of further debate and research into the past and present cultural practices of rearing children, and how this was perceived by different societies (James and Prout, 2004).

More recently, we have seen discussions about the nature of children and childhood taking place at national levels, with the areas of law, policy, and medicine being particularly prominent in this regard (*ibid.*). In the second half of the twentieth century, we also saw the emergence of an additional argument that childhood is a comparatively recent phenomenon, as there is little evidence of its existence pre-dating the Renaissance (Boas, 1966; Ariès, 1962; Postman, 1994). Defining contemporary childhood has been anything but straightforward.

Yet despite such attempts to pin the word down in terms of its deeper significance within society, an overview of the wider literature suggests that there is no real consensus about what childhood is supposed to be. This is in spite of such an extensive and prolonged collective interest in establishing its boundaries, or charting its beginning as a social construction, as outlined above. In admitting the complexity of the issue, many authors go on to define the absence of any consensus as a social problem in its own right (Buckingham, 2000; Louv, 2005; Palmer, 2006; Postman, 1994; Steinberg and Kincheloe, 2004; Zornado, 2001). Without a consensus, they argue, there can be no true identity for the child. And without a true identity, we are unable to rear children properly. In some cases, authors predict nothing less than social catastrophe, with their books bearing emotive titles such as *Toxic Childhood* (Palmer, 2006) and *Last Child in the Woods* (Louv, 2005). To an extent our own provocative title for this book – *Invisibly Blighted* – also reflects this position.

However if we examine literature relating to the history of childhood carefully, we can see some recurrent themes emerging, which arguably *are* collectively understood to some degree. Constructions of childhood can usefully be categorized according to these themes. The nature of how this is done is dependent on the period of history under scrutiny, the social context of children's upbringing, and the geographical region in which they lived (Cunningham, 1995). The primary themes that emerge recurrently within the literature are as follows:

Biological

This category refers to a dominant discourse surrounding child physicality. Within this discourse, children are seen as physically immature in comparison with adults, which can lead to vulnerability, for example on grounds of size, weight, or disease resilience (Pinchbeck and Hewitt, 1969; Cleverley and Phillips, 1986; James and Prout, 2004). It can also bring about 'coddling' and concern for aspects of the child's existence such as health and hygiene (Ariès, 1962).

We explore this category in depth in Chapters 4 and 5 by examining recent phenomena such as websex[1] and sexting[2]. These activities demonstrate a tension between children's perceived physical and emotional maturity, and their interactions with technology, suggesting that adult preconceptions about the biological basis for childhood amongst schoolchildren are being challenged. We look at the technologies that children have access to through their own volition, and the potential future impact that this may have on high risk and criminal behaviour. We also address issues such as early exposure to sexual content, sexting for coercion, and normalized attitudes to what one might consider to be harassment in offline contexts.

Developmental

Within this model of childhood, children are engaged in an ongoing process of learning and development, which may be initiated by themselves, or which may be more formal (Locke, 1693; Rousseau, 1762; Piaget and Inhelder, 1969; Brown, 2002).[3] Within this theme, there are different conceptualizations of learning. For example, Locke described the child as a *tabula rasa* or blank slate, upon which learning could be written, whereas Rousseau defined children as 'natural' and needing 'denaturing' in order for them to join with the rest of society.

In the light of these philosophical and psychological positions, in Chapter 3 we discuss how children's social attributes and learning are measured, and the impact that this has on perceptions of the role and function of schooling within contemporary society. We also discuss how tracking children's social identity and development can become a commodity in its own right, and the consequences of this for children's information privacy as they develop into adults. This is also addressed in Chapter 2, where we look at the sociology of risk in relation to children, and consider the relationship between conceptualizations of risk, and statistical risk, aspects that are frequently in conflict in contemporary society.

Moral

Children are seen as being unable in some situations to take responsibility for their own actions, which may be rooted in religious doctrine, and in some cases may be considered to require punishment (Greven, 1991; Bunge, 2001).[4] They are also sometimes classed as innocents (Calvert, 1992; Higonnet, 1998; Meyer, 2007), or inspiring dangerous erotic attraction (Kincaid, 1992). Throughout this book, we develop thinking about children and morality in various ways by exploring recent shifts in social mores related to social networking, sexuality, and children's interpersonal relationships. We also discuss the role of state monitoring of children's social and learning outcomes, with the child's privacy sometimes being seen as subservient to the needs of the state in terms of schooling, welfare support, and healthcare, and child protection being invoked as grounds for this.

The child protection environment is discussed in more depth in Chapter 4. In this chapter, we report the findings of the 360 Degree Safe self-review tool for schools, which allows them to analyse their work in developing safe online behaviours. We argue that in the light of our study, the UK education system is not currently equipped to address questions, issues, and concerns arising from a hyper-connected, unregulated childhood.

Consumerist

Children are positioned within a marketized model of childhood, in which consumer goods such as toys both reflect and determine modes of existence (Cannella and Kincheloe, 2002; Steinberg and Kincheloe, 2004; Postman, 1994; Zornado, 2001; Cross, 1997). This can result in a hyperreality, where the socially constructed version of childhood is exaggerated and consequently replaces the real thing (Steinberg and Kincheloe, 2004). This may be perceived as harmful (Buckingham, 2000; Postman, 1994; Palmer, 2006) or having the effect of disempowering children (Formanek-Brunell, 1993).

Childhood and the technological age

By categorizing constructions of childhood in this way, we start to see how childhood fits within a highly technological society, and where the fault lines might be. Within the categories described above, the most significant fault line appears to be between children and consumerism, which is the category that dominates public debate most frequently. This dominance can be attributed to the increased availability of disposable income and mass-produced goods, combined with the growth of the mass media and internet and a mechanism for promoting and facilitating unregulated uptake. Parents and children form a ready-made market within this type of society and in doing so, contribute to economic growth (Furnham and Gunter, 1998). In turn, this extensive engagement is argued to have contributed to a general decline in moral responsibility (Doyle, 2009), which we see impacting on children's use of technology and their exposure to extreme violence and sexuality online.

Such a decline is a justifiable concern. For example, in developing a consumerist approach to defining childhood, we risk distilling a highly idealized view of what childhood means, as a result of the hyperreality described earlier in this chapter. This can manifest itself in different ways. For example, much has been written recently about the 'pinkification' of clothes and toys, with many products now specifically aimed at girls, contributing to an increasing gender divide (Paoletti, 2012; Martinson, 2011). Similarly, the apparent dominance of football and sport as desirable masculine interests brings with it a structure for male behaviour as boys learn to navigate possible identities (Swain, 2000). This risks increasing gender inequality, and with it, reducing personal empowerment and diminishing a sense of personal agency. We see this reinforced in the virtual and connected worlds inhabited by many children.

In this way, therefore, children and their identities themselves are effectively commoditized, and families defined through what Pugh has described as 'child rearing consumption' (Pugh, 2009). The toys and outfits they buy for their children, and the moral framework in which this is justified within the family as well as to the external world, all act as indicators of status and personal values. In this book, we show how this is extrapolated out to the online environment their children experience. We have found in our research that whether parents supervise their children's online interactions closely can be seen as a function of social class and parenting skill. Similarly parental willingness to invest in certain types of hardware, or paid subscriptions to internet forums, or smartphones, can have an effect on the type of virtual worlds their children encounter, and what type of digital life they are able to experience. You are what you buy.

This commodification of all aspects of childhood, and drive for status, is not confined to families. The existence of a technology-led audit culture has also made data concerning children and their school performance increasingly valuable. Data are even potentially saleable to commercial organizations, a step which is currently being considered by the UK Government. This use of data impacts on the branding and marketing of children's schools, with the extensive collection of data being a significant concern, also used as a proxy for efficiency and professionalism. Given the role of school choice within a marketized education economy, this plays an increasingly significant role in the definition of childhood, the understanding of age-related norms, as well as the expectations and status surrounding different child identities.

Changing childhood

It is clear that, all too often, we look at childhood exclusively through the lens of adulthood, without necessarily being fully aware of the implications of doing so. The growth of the internet has played a part in this, as children's experience of the world is no longer curated by parents and teachers in the way it might have been in previous years. Children have been propelled into a new social space attendant with its own new opportunities and risks. In the light of all of these issues, and their underlying philosophies, our book examines the role information technologies play in creating and sustaining such tensions, as well as the role of schools and related organizations in feeding the status quo. Only by laying this out for debate can society move towards a more appropriate definition of childhood for the twenty-first century.

Notes

[1] To engage in sexual activity over webcam with a partner of either sex.

[2] Sexting is the act of sending sexually explicit text messages back and forth with a partner.

[3] This may include digital images. Calvert offers a simplified historic classification of shifts in childhood along these lines, with the 'inchoate adult' being the usual view from 1600–1750, the 'natural child' described by Rousseau dominant from 1750–1830, and the concept of the 'innocent child' coming to the fore from 1830–1900 (Calvert, 1992).

[4] The impact of this on law is interesting. In the UK, the age of criminal responsibility is 10, for example. Between the ages of 10 and 14 the prosecution can make the case that children were aware they were committing a serious crime. After the age of 14, they are held to be fully responsible for their actions in the same way as an adult. It should be noted that in the tenth century the age of responsibility was originally 12, but after consultation this changed to 15. As Cunningham shows, the age of criminal responsibility has not changed much over the centuries (Cunningham, 1995).

Chapter 2

How risky is it to be a child? Towards a sociology of uncertainty

The idea of being worried about child safety is nothing new. Nothing is more emotive than reports of children being involved in crime, accidents, and disaster. Whether it is iconic photos of burned children from the Vietnam War from 1972; the chilling 1973 UK public information film 'Lonely Water', which discouraged young people from swimming in rivers; reports of children escaping from the 2004 school siege at Beslan; or pictures of a drowned Syrian toddler lying on a Turkish beach in 2015; we are neurologically hard-wired to become upset about such things. Protecting children is central to the human condition, and for that reason, we give a great deal of conscious and subconscious thought to how we look after our young. Intrinsic within this is a daily attempt to keep them safe, and this means regularly assessing risk. However as a society, risk is not something we find it easy to assess.

The reason for this is that risk is a social construction, particularly in relation to children. We know this because it is clear that conceptualizations of childhood have changed over the centuries, and with them, associated perceptions of risk. For example, where children may have been able to roam for miles around their homes in the past, the geographical space they are allowed to occupy shrank considerably over a period of six decades, and presumably continues to do so (Mey and Günther, 2014; Hillman *et al.*, 1988; Saracho and Spodek, 1998). In addition, while the main peril for some children may once have been considered spiritual, for example failing to be baptized before falling prey to an untimely death (Schofield and Midi Berry, 1971), since the decline of religious practice and the advent of vaccinations and antibiotics, most parents of children in industrialized nations today would no doubt say that they feel a reasonably good sense of control and agency with regard to their children's health. This is in contrast to the situation of children living in low-income economies who face real threats to their survival such as war, famine, illness, infectious disease, and vulnerability to natural disasters such as earthquakes, flooding, and drought.

It is clear that for those growing up in an industrialized country, it has probably never been safer to be a child, yet it seems we still feel the need to find aspects of risk to worry about. To that end, the twenty-first century has brought with it new and increased concerns, amplified by social and mass media reporting. Such a tendency is sometimes classified as a 'moral panic' in the research literature.[1] Within this framework of moral panic, risks commonly invoked range from frequent, low-risk events such as minor food hygiene or bullying problems, to infrequent, high-risk events such as paedophilia-related crime, fires, terrorist attacks, and serious adverse weather events. Within these parameters, schools are expected to engage in resilience planning to ensure the safety of pupils within their charge. Yet because of the socially constructed nature of risk, this is something that must be done with one eye on public relations and the media. This makes proper risk assessment more difficult and potentially less effective than it needs to be.

This chapter argues that there is a need for more sociology to be done in explaining the nature of children's risk within contemporary society. If risk is classified as a social problem, it is easier to explore why what we might term *moral panic* (Cohen, 2002) has arisen, and how it might be possible to move forwards. To this end, there are several themes that deserve particular attention. Firstly, examining definitions of risk is a useful starting point. Then it is helpful to examine the apparently paradoxical rise in risk and disaster management policies at a time when the idea of the expert is subject to increasing mistrust (Urry, 2003). An understanding of power relationships in times of what might be perceived as a kind of existential *collective stress* (Barton, 1969) plays an important role here as well. Finally, it is useful to examine the desire of individuals for a sense of personal and collective agency in the face of adverse events, something we see represented in the language of risk and a particular *Weltanschauung* or world view adopted by certain groups. This is underpinned by the desire for collective sense-making and/or a genuine fear of becoming victims. All of these considerations are useful in helping identify the influences that are shaping risk perception in relation to children in twenty-first-century Western Europe as well as the US and other countries. In this chapter, these themes are considered in the light of the probability of different events as well as their likely seriousness. The primary focus is on examples from the UK, which we consider to provide a particularly extreme case study of collective parental anxiety regarding risk, but we draw on international examples where possible.

It is clear that there are several key factors that are influencing risk assessment in a way that is unrelated from the statistical probability of serious harm. These factors include the role of power and vested interests in maintaining a rhetoric of crisis (for example, safety compliance as a professional currency). Another factor is the impact of the internet in speeding up perceptions of time, compressing distance, and increasing the perception of event frequency, giving a sense of something the social anthropologist Lévi-Strauss might call a 'hot chronology' (Lévi-Strauss, 1994). Anxieties regarding the increasing complexity of society are often conflated with these factors, leading to real concern on the part of families and teachers as they seek to navigate a realistic and sensible path, what Backett-Milburn and Harden (2004: 431) describe as 'the shifting and dynamic nature of the mundane negotiation of risk'. We argue for a more sophisticated twenty-first-century debate about the nature of risk and what we are prepared to tolerate for our children.

Creating definitions of risk – a difficult task

As discussed in the introduction, there are no fixed definitions available for the notion of risk. Many writers including Quarantelli (1998), Giddens (1991), and Beck (2007) have made this point repeatedly. Risk can also be seen as distinct from the idea of disaster or catastrophe. As Beck writes:

> Risk is not synonymous with catastrophe. Risk means the anticipation of catastrophe. Risks concern the possibility of future occurrences and developments; they make present a state of the world that does not (yet) exist. Whereas every catastrophe is spatially, temporally and socially determined, the anticipation of catastrophe lacks any spatio-temporal or social concreteness.
>
> (*ibid.*: 9)

Therefore one way of seeing risk is that it is a relatively fluid concept that depends on context for its meaning. This is primarily because tolerance for risk has changed throughout history. One example of this change is the way that the distance children can roam from home has reduced. In the 1930s, the work of German researcher Martha Muchow painted a picture of a social world in which children were able to engage with and appropriate urban space independently, reshaping it into ersatz playgrounds to suit their needs (Mey and Günther, 2014). This was a world in which children were actively encouraged to leave the home on sunny days in search of both formal playgrounds, and informal, improvised play opportunities on waste ground and so on, walking much further from home without parents than we might expect them to in the twenty-first century. The ability of relatively young children to experience this level of independence subsequently reduced over time, and unaccompanied young children have now more or less disappeared from twenty-first-century urban streets in many situations. This has been quantified in various studies. For example, in research by public health physician William Bird (reported in Souter-Brown, 2014), we see that over the course of four generations, roughly a century, the permitted roaming space available to an eight-year-old boy shrank from six miles for a great-grandfather, to one mile for a grandfather, to half a mile for a mother, and then finally for a contemporary eight-year-old living in the same location as his forebears, a mere 300 metres from his house.

The restriction in movement is not necessarily a function of traffic density, as is often argued. As Hillman *et al.* (1988) make clear, between 1922 and 1986, roads in Britain were described as increasingly safe, due to reducing casualties. Yet a factor in defining them as safe is that in many cases, pedestrians and cyclists have simply stopped using them freely, leading to apparent reductions in child road deaths per 100,000 children that doesn't reflect the reality of children's lives. In the same report, Hillman *et al.* report that parents cited molestation more frequently than traffic as grounds for curtailing permission for children to be out after dark, even though the likelihood of an averse 'stranger danger' event in this regard is very small indeed (Pritchard *et al.*, 2013). Hillman *et al.* describe the attitude of German parents during the same period to be more accepting of risk, despite the comparative environmental situations being broadly similar. Clearly, therefore, the relationship between risk, danger, safety, and parental perception is a complex one here and poorly grounded in the statistical measures available.

At the other end of the scale in terms of parental anxiety lies the concept of the 'disaster' (or catastrophe, as Beck might label it), which may take various forms. This could mean a natural disaster such as a flood or earthquake, a health disaster such as a disease epidemic, a terrorist attack, a large-scale accident such as a train or aeroplane crash, or something similar. For parents in the 1970s and 1980s this may even have meant a nuclear event. All these things are considerably less likely to happen than an individual child being knocked off a bike by a car, for example, but the unpredictability, severity, and scale of disasters means that they represent our most fundamental human fears in relation to our own survival. Even here definitions can be elusive, however. How do we differentiate between something that is just difficult to cope with, and something that represents a threat to survival? Up front they may look familiar to those caught up in the situation, and sometimes it is only with the benefit of hindsight that we are able to give an event a sense of scale and proportion and label it accordingly.

Bearing this perceptual difficulty in mind, sociologists of disaster document how people behave during periods of *collective stress* (a term coined by Barton, 1969) and here it is clear that different models exist when defining the scale and severity of a disaster (Dombrowsky, 1989; 1998). It may be that it makes sense to look at numbers injured or dead (something that could be described as an insurance model). Another useful classification tool might be a lack of nutrition/clothing/housing/aid (something that might be described as a Red Cross model). A third classification might be the breakdown of public order and safety (something that could be described as a government model). In addition to Dombrowky's useful list of classifications, the psychological impact of disaster may also be significant, and the role of time, space, and severity is also likely to be a factor (Sorokin and Merton, 1937).

Within such models, while we see the effect of events on the human race as a whole, a full understanding of the perception of risk and disaster in the context of children needs to go beyond this, and beyond the kinds of cataclysmic natural or war-related disasters we might see on news services. Alternatively if we simply rely on published statistical information about children's risk and associated reports, we reduce the framework down to a focus on medical and traffic-related issues, as little alternative work is done on risk in other areas for children (as opposed to humans in general). This means we need to move beyond the aetiology of disaster, as listed above, towards a more subjective view that allows us to consider the lived experience of risk by children and those around them.

To explore this properly we can borrow from Urry's 'Five Elements model' (Urry, 2003) and apply this to the particular situation of children. Urry came up with five general categories that can be used to understand disaster by allowing us to understand more about processes that unsettle people, including aspects of uncertainty and the loss of ability to define a situation. These five categories are:

- Structure
- Flow
- Ideology
- Performance
- Complexity.

In the next section we explore these categories in relation to children and risk/disaster, and their perception within society.

Structure

While Giddens (1991) sees childhood as what he might call a 'sequestered' social state, with childhood having been moved from the public to a private, domestic domain, we also live in a time where attendance at school allows the state to place children in cohorts, and determine what is normal or not normal for children at different ages. This gives the relationship between home, school, and social policy a certain interconnectedness, which brings with it in turn pressure for parents to conform. Within this is a sense of what is appropriate in terms of risk. Therefore if one set of parents decides it is appropriate for a child to cycle to school from the age of nine, and all the other local parents decide it is not, the child cyclist will be seen as some kind of risk 'outlier' and indeed one can even imagine a situation where a parent might be spoken to by the school and informed that their actions are unusual in permitting this. In this way, anxiety levels are potentially raised by the structural situation of the environment external to the child. An additional factor here is immediacy. The nature of mass media and social media in the digital age means that space and time are compressed. In this climate, news feels like it is happening on the doorstep, and happening all the time. The consequence of this is that urban risk factors are routinely applied to rural situations inappropriately, for example the concept of 'stranger danger' being used to discourage children from interacting with unknown adults, whereas in smaller communities this may be helpful or even necessary for a child's well-being. Similarly the fear of road traffic accidents may lead indirectly to child obesity as children are increasingly driven long distances rather than walking or cycling.[2] In this category, external social structures are therefore used to give an indication of perceived risk and promote particular types of conformity.

Flow

In the previous section we touched on the influence of mass media and social media on perceptions of risk. In this category of flow, we see the role of charities, government departments, and non-governmental organizations seeking to influence the social environment of children via harnessing the flow of information. For example, the UK's National Society for the Prevention of Cruelty to Children (NSPCC) ran a Green Dot/Full Stop campaign, which ended in 2008. The NSPCC engaged firms such as leading advertising agency Saatchi and Saatchi to create headlines such as 'Together we can stop child abuse. FULL STOP'. This campaign eventually raised £250m for the charity and made the issue of child abuse more prominent in the public consciousness. However the charity has been heavily criticized for spending disproportionately on advertising to the tune of approximately half its revenue (*Daily Telegraph*, 2003), and similarly criticized for invoking child safeguarding issues inappropriately to engender a sense of moral panic and encourage even higher levels of fundraising from the general public (Furedi, 2014).

This media-friendly approach is similar to the United Nations Children's Fund (UNICEF). This charity was originally set up to provide for the physical survival of children after the Second World War, but subsequently repositioned by Chief Executive Carol Bellamy (a former US corporate lawyer and financier) to emphasize advocacy for children's rights rather than maintaining a primary focus on child mortality. This new focus was clearly visible in their 2005 report, which asked why millions of children were 'losing out on their childhood' (UNICEF, 2005). This repositioning was subject to extensive criticism by the medical profession amongst others. As Horton (2004) argued:

> A preoccupation with rights ignores the fact that children will have no opportunity for development at all unless they survive. The language of rights means little to a child stillborn, an infant dying in pain from pneumonia, or a child desiccated by famine. The most fundamental right of all is the right to survive. Child survival must sit at the core of UNICEF's advocacy and country work. Currently, and shamefully, it does not.
>
> (*ibid.*: 2072)

There are two aspects to this. Individual organizations such as the NSPCC and UNICEF frequently seek to harness the flow of information in this way, and in doing so, extend the range and involvement of their activities in the child protection/safeguarding/rights sector, leading to the identification of issues that they can appropriate as campaigns to bring to the public attention. This is always well-intentioned: after all, who would disagree with the need to protect children or give them rights? However the second aspect is that there are invariably unintended consequences as a result of doing this, because of the identification of such campaigns on the grounds of being (a) simple to articulate to the public, and (b) apparently possible to do something about. This can distort the severity and scale of a problem in the eye of the public. In doing this, it has the effect of changing the perception of particular kinds of risk, in this case privileging child abuse as a cause at the expense of social deprivation, and children's rights at the expense of poverty, disease, and starvation, both of which are significantly more likely to kill children (Pritchard *et al.*, 2013; Horton, 2004).

Ideology

As we have argued throughout this chapter, risk is not just about actual likelihood, but also about belief, and it is in the category of ideology that we see the paradoxical situation of a desire to protect children increasing other risks. As Hillman *et al.* make clear, driving a child to school increases the likelihood of road traffic accidents for other children who are not in a car. Similarly, a professionalized rhetoric of risk can override individual judgements via unintended consequences. A good example of this was the way many UK schools reacted to the rise of digital photography at school events. Many parents were unfairly prohibited from taking pictures of their own children in the name of child protection/safeguarding by head teachers, who freely invoked the Data Protection Act (1998) as grounds for any prohibition. However a school play or concert is considered to be a private event in UK law and as such the Data Protection Act (DPA) does not apply here. In other words, parents do not need permission from the school in order to take digital photographs for private use. At the same time, schools were routinely using digital photographs of children in publicity materials without parental permission, and also starting to collect biometric data without parental permission, for lunch payment purposes as well as library book loans. This did breach the DPA, but schools were frequently unaware of the anomaly. For this reason the Information Commissioner's Office had to issue guidance on taking photographs in schools (ICO, 2015), something we discuss in Chapter 3, on identity, and biometrics.

Another example of policy being lost in translation is the trend towards public leisure centres introducing strict parent:child ratios for public swimming sessions. These are a characteristic of the UK leisure industry as many fewer rules appear to exist for swimming pool parent:child ratios in the rest of Western Europe, where it is generally left up to parents to decide about appropriate balances. The UK ratios are rooted in guidance issued by the Institute of Sport and Recreation Management, but this is not always applied sensitively in practice (RoSPA, 2015). As a consequence, such ratios can be very complex for parents to navigate, and there is little if any flexibility. For example, taking the first result that appears in an internet search, we find the Tandridge Trust website, where there is a complex grid representing 12 different permutations of leisure centre (they run four facilities), sessions, age, and ratio, that users are required to navigate. In one box on the grid, for example, we learn that:

> All Gentle Splash and under-8s sessions have a ratio of 1 adult
> to 2 children under 4. All children under 4 are required to wear

a swim aid unless they are being supervised on a 1:1 basis. The ratio for 4–7 is 1:3 during these sessions.

(Tandridge Trust, 2015)

This statement is typical of other leisure centres across the country. The unintended consequence of rigid ratios such as these may be that parents are indirectly prevented from teaching their children to swim, if they feel unwelcome or wrong-footed by the leisure centre administrators, and discouraged from attending. Here we have an example of the legitimacy of a professional elite (leisure centre managers) assumed, and parents effectively disenfranchised in the process. This is also an example of risk-related decisions being highly bureaucratized in a manner previously described by Scott *et al.* (1998), standardizing responses without taking into account social context or life experience. An ideology of risk (relating to ratios) has overruled parental judgement. However, this was not the intention of the original guidance. As the UK's Royal Society for the Prevention of Accidents states:

The Institute of Sport and Recreation Management (ISRM) have guidance on this and many pool managers will use this guidance. Some parents have found the standard ratio of adults to children advised by the ISRM and used by pool managers, to be restrictive. The guidance issued by the ISRM does allow for flexibility based on the risk present at individual pools so it is worth discussing this with your local pool.

(Royal Society for the Prevention of Accidents, 2014)

Tracing the policy back to accident data, if we look at the swimming pool accident data for 2013,[3] for example, we see that death by drowning in swimming pools for children is extremely rare, with just six adults and children dying in swimming pools in the UK, of whom three were children (RoSPA, 2014). If we look more closely at the data, this includes incidences where an adult or child died because of a heart attack in the water, for example, so might have died anyway. The data also do not distinguish between privately owned swimming pools, hotel pools (where lifeguards are not usually present), and publicly owned leisure centres (where lifeguards are always present). So we don't know exactly how many children died in a leisure centre swimming pool in 2013, and what the relationship was to the type and quantity of supervision. More worryingly, the consequence of ratio policies may simply be to defer deaths, in the manner that Hillman *et al.* reported for road traffic accidents: the heavily supervised young children of today may simply be more likely to drown as youths because they don't go swimming very often and their water safety awareness is comparatively low, compared to that of children who swim frequently under less supervision. If we look at the data for swimming in rivers, we see that the figure for older children is indeed higher, in that 15 young people between the ages of 15–19 drowned, compared to only one in a swimming pool, suggesting risks are being taken outside the context of leisure centres, resulting in fatalities. This may be because lifeguards are very good at saving lives (which we do not doubt they are), or it may also be because young people are not sufficiently safety conscious when unsupervised (which we suspect is also a significant factor). Either way, it is reasonable to wonder whether deaths are simply being deferred. In this context, ideology does not always align with statistical risk. In comparison, in the US the issue of children's swimming risk has been approached more scientifically, with a greater emphasis on the public health aspects of mortality at a population level. There has been more sophisticated analysis of the nuances of risk, and several papers have pointed to the additional risks faced by foreign-born males and black males, putting forward tentative explanations for this (Saluja *et al.*, 2006; Brenner *et al.*, 2001). Unlike the UK, research attention seems to be focused on areas of actual, rather than perceived, risk.

Given that there can be a mismatch between the perception of risk in this regard, and the reality of what is happening statistically, it is helpful to give some consideration to underpinning reasons. One significant factor is likely to be changes to the legal system. In 1995, for example, the UK Government introduced the possibility of Conditional (No Win No Fee) agreements in personal injury cases. This was aimed at widening access to justice whilst also reducing the burden on the state. However this change led to a significant increase in the volume of personal injury cases (Association of British Insurers, 2012), which may have been influenced by the ability of personal injury lawyers to advertise their services. This is not simply a UK issue. For example, across Europe there has been a statistical reduction in accident-related deaths with a corresponding increase in personal injury compensation claims, although financial remedy varies a great deal amongst different member states, which has led to demands for reform (Vismara, 2014). It is mirrored in the United States where there have been similar demands to address the substantial increase in personal injury cases since the 1950s. This type of legal action has sometimes been described as predatory, and it may have had the indirect effect of stifling innovation amongst manufacturers and entrepreneurs (Graham *et al.*, 1991). If this is the case, we see an example of ideology at work here, where a financially motivated risk aversion process has taken place. To paraphrase Douglas and Wildavsky (1983), as we become richer we can afford to become more cautious.

Performance

So far in this chapter we have focused on the notion of relatively small-scale risk negotiated by families and their immediate neighbourhoods. However if we move towards the notion of 'disaster', we see that there is potential for global interests both to define and magnify conceptualizations of risk. For example, the role of climate change on resilience planning is becoming increasingly significant, and international agreements are likely to rise in frequency and significance. This may result in international policies coming into conflict with local, more parochial concerns. For example, we have already stated in this chapter that it is likely to be more risky to walk or cycle to school than to be driven, if the majority of children are being driven. The carbon footprint of such risk-related behaviour is such that it may contribute to even higher, more serious risks for children in the medium to long term, including changes to weather systems. In another sense, however, it is important for the disaster rhetoric of climate change to grow, as invoking a global problem is likely to have the effect of unlocking resources for change. The same can be said to apply to issues such as child molestation, terrorism, and border control problems. The counterpoint to this is that, in each case, global communication systems are amplifying the effect of incidents. This means something that might previously have been regarded as regional in nature is conflated with larger international issues, giving the impression of a crisis of some kind, when this might in fact represent relatively isolated incidents that were always evident throughout society, only now they have become defined as issues. This leads to what Beck terms the 'staged anticipation of disasters and catastrophes' (Beck, 2007: 11) in which governments and individuals are obliged to take preventative action, whether or not the risk has grown in any quantifiable sense (child molestation perhaps representing the best example of this). In this way we see risk as a form of policy performance.

Complexity

Giddens describes the ideal state being sought by citizens as a 'state of bodily and psychic ease' (Giddens, 1991) which is located in a relatively secure and predictable *Umwelt*, or in other words, the familiar physical and social environment of an individual. However disruption to the *Umwelt*, perhaps on account of the performance or staging of risk described in the previous section, can lead to shifts in the power balance between citizen and the authorities as citizens are rendered governable in the context of any changes.

We have already discussed the example of UK authorities imposing parent:child swimming ratios with little supporting empirical evidence, but a better example here is the struggle in the UK surrounding the introduction of Criminal Records Bureau (CRB) checks (operational 2003–12) and later the Vetting and Barring Scheme (operational but not fully live 2009–10) which had an even wider reach, the ContactPoint database (operational but not fully live 2007–10), criticized widely as being overly intrusive, and the current Disclosure and Barring Scheme (operational 2012 onwards). In this case, the original CRB scheme came in during 2003 in the aftermath of a double child murder. It then escalated in scale and reach over subsequent years, resulted in tens of millions of not just teachers and health workers, but also ancillary workers, volunteers, charity workers, and parents being screened for routine contact with children, even when this was to be in the presence of other adults.

All this came about from a desire to reframe the staging of risk in relation to children, with a view to preventing future crimes of child abuse and murder. In doing so, it appeared to promote a view that there was such a thing as an *ideal type* of vetted citizen, who was assumed to represent reduced risk in relation to contact with children. Clearly it could never offer any such assurance, involving only a retrospective view of the behaviour of any individual in relation to one aspect of their conduct within society (i.e. recorded criminal convictions from England). Yet there were a number of unintended consequences as a result of this policy, of which the most significant was the attitude of mistrust that it engendered throughout society. Amongst other things, adult men became increasingly reluctant to come forward to assist children, with this being seen as a 'state-sponsored activity' requiring official approval (Beckford, 2012). Obviously the complexity of rendering adults governable in this regard, and indeed to some extent alienated, had not been fully appreciated by the government, in its desire to be seen to be responsive and proactive. In failing to understand such complexity, the policy is likely to have had the effect of reducing the number of non-family members able and willing to support children in everyday life, paradoxically and presumably increasing various risks to children's well-being.

Towards a sociology of uncertainty

As discussed at the beginning of this chapter, the situation of children in relation to risk is particularly emotive, and this leads to people trying to make sense of things based on media reports and government guidance, whether or not either of these has any statistical basis in fact. As we have seen, in the confusion there is significant scope for a particular *Weltanschauung* or world view based on a set of assumptions that are not always relevant.

While we have been comparatively critical of a number of organizations in this regard, the real life context of their policies needs to be taken into account before judging them too harshly. Policymaking takes place in a society that has become increasingly disorientated with regard to its conceptualization of the role, function, and identity of children within it. Throughout each of the Five Elements we have worked through here, we see a particular reaction to perceived change in type and scale of risk for children that can frequently be termed a *moral panic,* because it does not necessarily correspond to any obvious increase in risk, only to an increased awareness of the occurrence of crime (for example, as a consequence of extensive reporting in the media).

The phrase 'moral panic' was coined in Stanley Cohen's 1972 book, and refers to a situation in which certain conditions or groups become defined as a threat to societal values and interests. In the introduction to the third edition (2002) Cohen presciently extends his definition to include child abuse, Satanic rituals, and paedophile registers as new forms of moral panic. Cohen emphasizes the role of the media in publicizing certain kinds of adverse events, ranging from accusations of Satanic abuse in the 1980s in Cleveland (*ibid.*: xv), to mobs marching on the houses of alleged paedophiles (*ibid.*: xvi), leading to serious consequences for public order. It appears that the apparent loss of the ability to define a risk-related situation amongst many individuals becomes acute when it is distilled into a collective response, leaving the government to achieve a difficult balancing act between reaction and guidance. As Cohen writes:

> Public figures had to express sympathy with the parents and share the moral revulsion but also distance themselves from the mob. This was easily done by repeating the inherently negative connotations of lynch mob and mob rule, the primitive atavistic forces whipped up by the *News of the World*. The rational polity is contrasted to the crowd: volative, uncontrollable and ready to explode.
>
> (*ibid.*: xvi)

Any difficulties in appraising risk for children are therefore rooted in the fact that risk has to be regarded as a social construct. Within this, the role of power is significant and there are notable vested interests in maintaining a rhetoric of risk/crisis. These vested interests include that of the tabloid newspaper that appropriates such a risk narrative in order to sell newspapers, the large IT company that tenders to develop and run a large-scale database to monitor individuals, and perhaps the charity executive looking to build a career through enhancing the relative status of a charity within society. All these stakeholders seek a tactical advantage in terms of commanding resources or attention. It is here where the term 'risk' is most widely deployed and even abused.

A key factor in this contemporary escalation of the children's risk narrative is likely to be the breakdown of trust in modern society. We live in a comparatively fragmented modern society, in the throes of a technological revolution. This has led to a desire for individual agency which is in conflict with a sense of loss of control. This makes us uncertain where to invest our trust, and particularly receptive to risk-related statements. Within this context we see safety compliance grow as a means of professional currency, as we saw in relation to swimming pools. We see a desire to rely on expert knowledge in conflict with desire for the democratization of knowledge, leading to mistrust of various forms of expertise, as we saw in relation to road traffic accident data and the risks of increased car journeys for children. These aspects of the modern risk narrative represent just two examples of conceptual shifting sands as society regroups, and risk moves from an objective to a subjective conceptualization.

In seeking to understand how risky it is to be a child, we need to be aware that the late twentieth and early twenty-first centuries have brought with them a very particular view of risk. This may well be out of step with actual statistical risk, so part of the role of the modern government, academics, and risk professionals should be to challenge this, in order to reassure individuals whilst promoting individual freedoms. Equally, those in positions of authority need to take responsibility for not over-stating risk in order to gain a tactical advantage in going about their business. Only then can we ensure our children are truly cared for in an appropriate and effective way.

A postscript

During the preparation of this chapter we came across an interesting example of conflicting risk assessment imperatives in practice. In preparation for an Office for Standards in Education (Ofsted) visit in 2015, a local primary school asked their children what is a fairly routine safeguarding question as part of a school attitudes survey: 'Do you feel safe at this school?' The response was mixed but overall it seemed that to many children the answer was 'No!' The children reported that there were two main problems with the school. The first was that there were many spiders and this was scary. The second was that they were convinced the building was haunted, and this felt even scarier. The moral of this tale is that we need to be very careful when imposing a twenty-first-century view of safeguarding on our children, who have legitimate concerns of their own that require attention.

Notes

[1] We define this term later in the chapter.

[2] Hillman *et al.* (1988) also came to various conclusions about the link between risk and reduction in walking and cycling by children but linked this to deferred deaths by young drivers. The implicit assumption in the report was that children were not becoming sufficiently familiar with road use. However their report predates what has since been described as the 'obesity epidemic'.

[3] There is no reason to think 2013 is atypical in terms of accident data so this is provided as an appropriate example.

Chapter 3

Identity and biometrics: Convenience at the cost of privacy in English schools

Surveillance technologies are always a lot more fun in the movies than in real life. In the 2002 Steven Spielberg film *Minority Report*, for example, there is an amusing scene where a couple obediently interrupts a heated domestic argument, so that little electronic spider robots can scan their irises to verify that they are not, in fact, Tom Cruise (who has just had an iris transplant in any case, specifically to avoid this scenario). This is fortunately not the experience for most twenty-first-century citizens, although biometrics are certainly much more widespread now than they were when the film was made. Positioning itself away from science fiction, this chapter explores the day-to-day reality of biometric use in English schools among children. It is clear that understanding of privacy issues is still in its infancy in many English schools. Biometrics are widely used, but while they are not properly understood, this also brings unexpected democratic consequences.

Children and biometric technologies

Using children's biometric data may sound cutting edge, but it is nothing new. To give a sense of historical perspective, children's handprints that form part of early cave paintings have been found dating from 35,000 years ago in France and Spain, where they represent some of the earliest examples of European Upper Palaeolithic cave art (Department of Archaeology, Durham University, 2012). More recently, the first officially recorded use of children's biometrics dates from fourteenth-century China, when Chinese merchants were allegedly stamping children's palm prints and footprints on paper with ink as a method of distinguishing individuals (Shoniregun and Crosier, 2008: 1). Since then, however, we have seen many changes in biometric techniques, as well as our tolerance for them.

One area where children's biometrics have recently been heavily used is in the area of education. Many English schools now use biometric technologies to track the routine interactions of children and their teachers with different school systems such as libraries and cafeterias. Indeed school biometrics have proved relatively popular with end users on grounds of convenience and affordability (Boyce *et al.*, 2010; Darroch, 2011) and consequently there has been enthusiastic uptake in England over the last decade. While there is no central record of where these systems are used, Darroch (*ibid.*) suggested that biometric systems had been adopted by 2,000 secondary schools, or 40 per cent of the total, as well as 2,000 primary schools, or 10 per cent of the total. By 2012/13, a series of systematic Freedom of Information Act requests suggested that approximately 866,000 English children in 2,500 schools were required to give their fingerprints in order to access the school canteen and library (Big Brother Watch, 2014). Clearly uptake of biometric systems amongst English schools is extensive. Yet there are a number of surprising aspects to its adoption, mainly technological and privacy related.

In a purely technological sense, biometric measures do not represent an ideal token for identifying the young. The basis for biometrics is that physical characteristics are converted into machine-readable code, which is then turned into a mathematical algorithm (varying from system to system) and stored on a database as an identification token for an individual. Biometrics can take a number of forms, including facial and iris scans, ear patterns, and fingerprints. More recently, systems have also been introduced that involve palm prints, gait analysis, and vein readings, as well as occasionally what are known as 'exotic' biometric measurements, including heartbeat recognition and voice recognition (Zhang, 2000). The biometric industry is predicated on the assumption that physical measures such as these are unique, determined at birth, and consistent throughout the life course. While this may to a large extent be true in adult life, it is not necessarily the case for children, and the accuracy of such systems has therefore been contested (Kindt, 2007: 166; McCahill and Finn, 2010). Depending on how a school chooses to set its software sensitivity settings, the 'False Accept' or 'False Reject' rates of fingerprints in a school situation is likely to be around 2.5 per cent. Put another way, in a school of 1,000 pupils, 25 of them are likely to have their fingerprints regularly confused by the system. Additionally, the platen (scanning device) itself commonly fails, requiring cleaning between uses, or rejecting fingerprints when they are the wrong temperature (Parziale, 2008). Yet despite these reliability problems, and alleged technical hurdles, we see that biometric measures are increasingly being used to track English children as they go about their daily lives.

This tracking of physical characteristics represents the rise of something that has become known as the 'audit culture' (Power, 1997; Strathern, 2000; Apple, 2010). In such a culture, minute variables relating to individuals are collected and analysed for a number of administrative and policy purposes. For many in society, this has become relatively inescapable, and something Hope (2007: 361) describes as the 'silent, continuous and automatic monitoring of an individual's everyday life'. In relation to biometrics in particular, others have described this as a 'post-panoptic era' (Deleuze, 1992; McCahill and Finn, 2010)[1] in which the body acts as a regulatory mechanism in place of self-regulation in behavioural terms. Your body becomes your password, determining whether you are allowed into a space or are able to take advantage of services such as school lunches. Van der Ploeg (1999) terms this use of the body as identification token as the 'informisation of the body'. This highly mechanized, highly regulated reality is the social environment to which many English children are now becoming conditioned (Dowty, 2008), and later in the chapter we argue that this resembles Baudrillard's concept of hyper-compliance (1983), in which children and young people are subjected to extensive measurement and surveillance, rendering their existence as citizens inauthentic (in other words, remote from reality and existing in a computer rather than in real life).

Such data-led surveillance, or 'dataveillance', as Clarke (1991) describes it, raises the related question of children's data privacy rights. Before 2012, consent was not always obtained explicitly from parents in advance of fingerprinting children. This was contrary to the wider European picture, being more in line with contemporary trends in the United States. This disjuncture with the rest of Europe did not seem to be of particular concern to the British Government at the time. As a consequence, the EU Working Party established by Article 29 of Directive 95/46/EU addressed the issue of such monitoring on several occasions, particularly with reference to the use of biometric data in the context of children attending school. It repeatedly asked for stringent adherence to the data protection principles set out in the 95/46/EU Directive, with particular reference to proportionality, as well as the security of stored data. This was seen by the working party as being a matter of considerable concern. Yet despite the country's comparatively exposed position at the forefront of child population surveillance via biometrics, the UK Government did little to address the issue until 2012. At this point, it updated the 'Protection of Biometric Information of School Children' section of the Protection of Freedoms Act (UK Government, 2012). This made it explicitly clear that a parental signature was required in order to collect biometric data from children: in other words, the government clarified that consent was now to be 'opt-in' rather than 'opt-out', as had happened in many cases previously. In addition, children were able to opt out even if their parents had already given consent. Here we see the first significant governmental steps towards acknowledging children's privacy rights in an unequivocal manner, rather than relying on the ICO to steer schools in a more general sense. With the 2012 Protection of Freedoms Act we therefore see a shift in policy emphasis. The situation has moved from a relatively laissez-faire attitude towards child surveillance under New Labour, to promoting legal compliance obligations under the post-2010 Coalition government. Nevertheless, extensive fingerprinting of children continues.

The matter of how school administrators had become complicit in widespread, digitized child surveillance – not always compliant with the law – merits examination. We begin with a brief history of school administration.

The automation of the school office

Universal schooling existed for 135 years in England before the introduction of biometrics, and schools managed to keep track of their pupils during that time, with a high degree of success. This included times of war and pupil mass evacuation from urban areas. At no stage did schools resort to fingerprinting in order to do this, although it was an available technology even then. It was not until the early 2000s that attitudes changed and fingerprinting technologies were adopted in schools. Conversely, in the rest of Europe, biometric measurements were invariably regarded with suspicion, as demonstrated by the EU Working Party concerns expressed above, and they were not used in schools. This highlights two important issues for consideration. Has adoption come about simply because of availability, or did biometrics answer a specific need in English schools, as opposed to those in other countries?

Looking at the first question above, it would be fair to argue that to a significant extent, supply led demand in the case of English schools. In the early 1990s we saw a fundamental shift from paper-based systems, with comparatively few identification categories, to electronic systems with significantly greater numbers of identification categories. This shift can be attributed to the vast expansion of computer processing power over the last two decades. This has led to increased affordability of complex digital systems, in turn presenting many new data collection opportunities for public and private sector organizations. The related development of hardware and software for such purposes has led rather than followed the needs of schools in this regard. There are two main contributory factors here:

1. Since the early 1990s, computer memory had grown exponentially and become significantly cheaper. The Acorn 3020 RISC-OS machine

typical of schools at that time might have had a total of 200 kilobytes of hard disk space, for example, and that hard disk space might have cost the school around £240 from a specialist supplier. In comparison, on Amazon at the time of writing we can purchase a generic 500 megabyte hard disk drive for £29.99 (so 2,500 times more hard disk memory space for 12.5 per cent of the cost). Such developments obviously meant that schools rapidly developed the ability to store more and more data over the past two decades.

2. Software packages were developed over the same period as a consequence of this enhanced storage capability, which allowed increasingly sophisticated manipulation of the data without high-level statistical or computer coding knowledge on the part of the user. For example, Microsoft Excel 5.0, launched in 1993, was readily available bundled with Microsoft Office, and allowed schools to automate many high-level analysis tasks. This could also be used in conjunction with Microsoft Access, one of the first mainstream database packages, launched in 1993. This introduced schools to the idea of populating particular fields with pupil data and then merging this into other software packages (such as Word or Excel, or school information management systems such as Capita's SIMS) as a means of processing data for different purposes.

In the context of school office automation, biometrics therefore lent themselves very well to the new database-orientated era of monitoring, being comparatively cheap and easy to implement: they could be used by schools in a straightforward manner for relatively low-level security functions.

Simplicity was only part of the story, however. Another factor in the widespread adoption of biometrics was the ability of schools to elect to buy such products without higher level authorization. This was rooted in the Local Management of Schools (LMS) policy that had been introduced as part of the UK's 1988 Education Reform Act. LMS meant that many budgetary powers were devolved to individual schools, and that schools were able to choose to invest in biometric systems comparatively easily as they came on to the market, without local and regional accountability being a significant issue for those responsible for procurement. In turn, the biometrics industry found schools to be a ready market for new products.

Additionally, during this period, many larger schools underwent significant investment, rebuilding, and remarketing under the aegis of the Building Schools for the Future (BSF) project, as well as being a consequence of the Academies policy. In the case of BSF, this was a government scheme where £55 billion was allocated to refurbish and upgrade the school estate nationally, as well as commissioning entirely new school buildings which were often oriented towards high levels of technology use. The scheme was axed by Secretary of State Michael Gove in 2010 after £5 billion had been spent. In the case of Academies, schools were frequently merged with other local schools, and/or taken over by educational organizations, with the aim of effecting rapid and highly visible school improvement via separation from Local Authorities and enhanced school autonomy (Curtis *et al.*, 2008). In both cases, rebranding the educational offer as being modernized and more aspirational was an important part of the process. In this context, biometric systems began to be seen as a proxy for indicating a modern, efficiently run learning environment and as a proxy for an idealized form of teacher professionalism (Selwyn, 2011; Boyce *et al.*, 2010).

The final factor in the extensive adoption of biometrics was that extensive and sometimes intrusive data collection practices were already in place in English schools, as previously outlined. Such data were collected in order to reduce administrative costs and streamline processes (for example, via the database package SIMS described earlier). In addition to any administrative function, these databases and others were also used to inform and develop government policy. To schools, it therefore seemed reasonable to add biometric information to the load, as the overall amount of children's personal data being collected at school levels and also nationally was already substantial. Table 3.1 gives an indication of the scale of this national pupil surveillance programme.

When adopting these extensive data collection technologies, there is little doubt that schools' intentions are benign. If we were to examine the copious institutional documents in existence explaining schools' reasoning for using high-level monitoring technologies, it is likely that we would see that the aim of such data collection practices is commonly put forward as one or more of the following:

1. A method of increasing public sector efficiency (for example, reducing the number of adults required to supervise children at school);
2. A means of effectiveness (for example, being able to track children's progress through the school in the short, medium, and long term);
3. A form of ensuring reliability (for example, being able to remedy any educational or administrative shortcomings of the school fairly rapidly);
4. A means of accountability (for example, being able to demonstrate to school inspectors that the school is functioning as it should); and
5. A means of ensuring confidentiality (for example, making it easier for children in receipt of Free School Meals to do so without classmates being aware).

Table 3.1: Large-scale English child data collection systems (1995 to date)

Name	Type	Nature of data	Access	Shared?
ContactPoint Live in 2009, database switched off 2010	Universal child database of all children in England and Wales	Unique identity number given at birth, plus personal details, and 'concerns' logged by health, education, and welfare professionals about children or their parents; youth offences; education; medical information	Social workers Police Head teachers Health professionals Education officials Government departments	Yes, with NHS Database and SureStart database
Police DNA database Live in 1995	DNA of 1.1 million children who have committed no offence	DNA	Police and law enforcement agencies	No
PLASC (Pupil Level Annual School Census) Began 1998, known as School Census since 2007, with data now collected three times a year	Information about all school pupils in England and Wales	Unique pupil number, personal information, educational programme followed, Special Educational Needs, deprivation measures, mother tongue, ethnicity, postcode	Schools Local authorities Education officials Researchers Government departments	Yes, with ContactPoint

Connexions Live in 2000	Information about pupils aged 14–19	Personal information; educational history; career information; financial status	Government departments, commercial organizations, schools, educational institutions	Yes, with ContactPoint
Ryogens (Risk of youth offending generic solutions) Live in 2003	Profiling tool for identifying children who may break the law in future	Personal details, checklist of risk factors flagged by professionals (e.g. frequently moving house, easily bored, poor general parenting skills)	Police, teachers, local authorities, healthcare professionals, social workers	No
SureStart Live in 1998	Details of children using SureStart service, and their families	Personal details, outcomes from using the service	Early years professionals	Yes, with ContactPoint
NHS Database Partially live in 2009	Health records	Personal details, electronic medical records	Health professionals	Yes, with ContactPoint
Vericool (internal to schools)	Commercial cashless and cardless registration and payment system	Biometric data (e.g. fingerprints), personal information	School administrators, head teachers	No

Arguably some or all of these motives might be regarded as reasonable. Clearly schools need to pay attention to pupil progress and be able to account for their practices to external bodies, to name two. However the very substantial level of data collection activity also raises serious questions about the nature of the data being captured and processed, the safeguarding procedures for doing so, as well as the implications for school administrators, pupils, and parents. Yet despite the extent of data collection taking place in UK schools, and the apparent risks to data privacy, research into the effect that this might have on pupils and teachers is in its infancy (Ashborne, 2000; Elliott *et al.*, 2004; Darroch, 2011). We now look at three early research studies that throw light on user attitudes towards biometrics in schools.

Identity and convenience

'Yeah, it's OK, because you want a book.'

The above quotation is from a 14-year-old child, taken from the final report of the Trustguide project (Lacohee *et al.*, 2006). This project was undertaken with two major technology providers, British Telecommunications PLC and Hewlett Packard. The motivation was to conduct a large qualitative study that would help service providers to understand public attitudes towards technology in order to improve provision, and therefore engagement between providers and consumers.

Within the project, we worked with children and young people in order to understand their attitudes towards online engagement. We carried out ten focus groups in four different schools, each involving fifteen young people between the ages of 14 and 16. While authentication technologies were included in the discussion guide for the focus groups, it should be noted that there was originally no plan to cover the subject of biometrics explicitly. However, in three of the schools where the focus groups took place, attendees volunteered opinions about the biometric systems used in their schools. Two types of system were discussed – cafeteria and library. Both had a similar approach, in that students were registered on the system and a scan of their thumbprint was taken and stored. Then when the students used the system (either to identify themselves to have a lunch purchase credited to them, or to take out a library book) they had their thumbprint scanned and they were authenticated via this biometric. In giving us this data, students were unexpectedly presenting us with one of the first pieces of research on attitudes towards biometrics in schools. The quotation at the beginning of this section is particularly apt, therefore, as it embodies a typical attitude encountered during the Trustguide project. In essence, we found that concerns about security and trust disappear when individuals are presented with something of personal benefit or convenience. The teenager in this case had not reflected on any concerns about the collection of his biometric information, because in his view, this system was 'good', as it meant he could take out books without having to remember his library card. Thus he was happy for his body to act as a medium for regulation in this instance, and effectively to be used as a password, as the only alternative apparently available to him required more effort on his part.

What was apparent from this work was that:

1. Children and young people had little opposition to the collection of their biometric data when it made life more convenient for them (i.e. being able to get lunch or withdraw a library book without some other token-based authentication system such as a card or password).
2. They had no idea where their data were stored, how long they were kept for, or who had access.
3. They had not really thought about the implications of this but, when it was discussed, did not really mind.

From the school staff perspective (as a result of follow-up interviews) similar attitudes were discovered:

1. Staff members viewed the systems as positive because it meant that pupils did not have to remember the lunch money, library card, etc.
2. In all the schools concerned, there was no policy in place to define access rights, duration of storage, physical and virtual security of any database, or the legal position around the storage of pupils' biometric data.
3. They had received no advice from the system vendor on the implications of storing young people's biometric data from a legislative or practice perspective.

This initial study had taken place in 2006, when these systems were very new and their introduction to schools was on an ad hoc basis (i.e. there was no regional or national guidance on the use of biometrics in schools whatsoever). In order to develop further data, a small case study was subsequently conducted in a primary school in 2011. In this study, an observational approach was used to understanding the attitudes of staff, vendors, and governors in procuring a new library system.

The motivation for the research was to determine whether, after five years of increased awareness raising (through organizations such as the Open Rights Group[2], No2ID[3], and LeaveThemKidsAlone[4]) and lobbying around the issues of fingerprinting in schools, there had been a change in attitudes and policy around biometric data. The study explored the experience of a school entering into a procurement process for a new library system. Throughout this process interviews were carried out with the head and chair of governors, a governors' meeting was attended and observed, and discussions were held with parents and pupils. The school in question was a small rural primary, with 70 pupils on roll; it had no policies related to data protection or online safety and ICT support was provided by an offsite company. If we compare it in profiling terms to the national 360 Degree Safe e-Safety database,[5] for example, it is typical of many small English primary schools in both composition and attitude towards data privacy in general.

As a result of the data collected, a number of observations around biometric data could be drawn:

1. The use of biometric data was viewed as a positive benefit in any new system – both the head teacher and chair of governors expressed their enthusiasm for a biometric system, as described by the vendor. They were reassured that the actual biometric for the child was not stored: instead an algorithm converted the print of each individual child into a unique number, and it would be this number that was stored, rather than the fingerprint image. However, when questioned neither could explain why this was 'better' in terms of data security or privacy.

2. The vendor provided no guidance whatsoever on security or data protection aspects of the system. It was proposed that the new system would be installed on a stand-alone PC in the school library – a publicly accessible area that was not monitored in any way. Aside from standard Windows authentication, accessed via a generic 'library user' login, there were no additional protection mechanisms on the machine. The school did not receive any advice on data protection legislation, whether biometric data needs to be more tightly controlled, or whether registration under the Data Protection Act was needed.

3. The school did not have a specific data protection policy as it was stated that this was not a statutory policy requirement and they came under their local authority's general data protection guidelines (which included nothing on biometrics and their storage).

4. The chair of governors, in particular, saw no problem at all from a social perspective with the collection of pupils' fingerprints. During the governors' meeting that was observed, she stated she had no problem with her children's fingerprints being collected (two of her own children

were at the school) because 'if you've done nothing wrong, what do you have to hide?' When pressed in the meeting on data access and storage duration, she said that she did not know.

5. Pupils at the school saw no problem with having their fingerprints taken – it was viewed as 'cool' by many and they also saw the benefit of not having to remember their library card. None saw any issues around data protection or who could access their fingerprints.

6. Parents were not aware of school's systems that collected fingerprint information and some were uncomfortable with the idea of their children's biometric information being collected. However, others saw no problem.

Clearly any system that requires authentication, in particular a system that involves some sort of financial transaction, benefits from the use of biometrics such as fingerprinting. This is because there is a comparatively low chance of denial of identity when taken from such a token, if the settings are fixed correctly. However, while technically the value of the biometric to administrators is clear, what is more concerning is that there is no consideration of the worth of this comparatively high-value biometric to the individual. Indeed, it seems as though it is being undervalued by being associated with something as mundane and everyday as the school cafeteria or library. This is particularly significant given the age of the individuals concerned, and the fact that their social identities are still being heavily influenced by the institution around them, namely school.

What was apparent is that there had been very little change in the development of advice for education establishments in the time between the two studies, from 2006–11. The issues that were identified from the Trustguide project were certainly reflected in the later case study and we were, once again, presented with a school that had little grasp of the sensitivity of biometric data or wider issues around data privacy. We acknowledge the discrepancy in group sizes and school sector between the two studies, and in particular the obvious sampling issues in the latter. However it is clear that the 2012 Protection of Freedoms Act was badly needed as a mechanism for making compliance issues explicit to all schools.

In the final study, we revisited some of the schools used in the original Trustguide study in the autumn term of 2015, to track once again how attitudes had changed over the course of nine years, and almost two complete cycles of pupils through the secondary phase of their school careers. We also wanted to establish whether the 2012 Protection of Freedoms Act, and associated clarification of parental consent issues, had led to changes in school processes. We spoke to six focus groups involving 38 pupils from Years 8 and 9, aged 12–14.

We found that adopting biometric systems in the schools had not been an unmitigated success. Two of the schools had retained their biometric lunch systems, but one had reverted to payment cards for lunch and the biometric system was viewed as a historic artefact experienced briefly by older siblings in years gone by. A third school had just adopted a biometric system. We found that pupils were not inducted into biometric systems in the same way that they had been in 2006 when such systems were relatively novel. There were no talks on the purpose of the system and related data privacy issues (indeed we found that data privacy was not mentioned at school much at all other than in the context of e-Safety). Instead, continued use was taken for granted in the schools that used them, and they also assumed that the pupils would be familiar with such systems.

It soon became clear that four key issues had arisen that may have contributed to all three schools and their pupils gradually becoming frustrated with the biometric systems they had bought into. These were:

1. Pupil resistance

Several pupils reported that 'people just walk past the device because there's a huge queue'. It was clear that biometric systems had not led to shorter lunch queues as initially promised by vendors, and frustrations at queuing had meant that some pupils were choosing not to pay for their meals, but instead bypassing biometric authentication equipment altogether and just helping themselves to food without paying. This also led to an enhancement in the social status of pupils who chose to break the rules. As one pupil pointed out, 'people think being bad is cool, so they want to get hold of free money'.

2. Pupil mistrust

Biometric systems were seen as unreliable. Typical comments were:

> 'Sometimes it doesn't work and you have to say your name and year';

> 'I put £5 on mine but then it was only showing £1.50 because someone else had been able to spend my money';

> 'I put money in my account and then other people put money in my account by accident as well'.

Many pupils reported issues with systems not reading their fingerprints properly, or losing money that they knew they had paid into their accounts and the money appearing in other pupils' accounts. From a technical point of view it would be fair to attribute these problems to the school's chosen False Acceptance/False Reject rate settings, in that clearly some pupils had similar digital identities to others and were experiencing regular and repeated problems accessing what was rightfully theirs, which caused annoyance and inconvenience. The school that had just adopted the biometric system seemed to experience the most problems and frustration in this respect. This also indicated that systems had not improved significantly since their initial adoption a decade previously.

3. Hygiene

Pupils repeatedly expressed disgust regarding the lack of hygiene surrounding biometric platen use. Comments included, 'I see loads of disgusting things on it', and 'Cards could be better because it's more hygienic'. Perhaps the most disturbing comment to the research team was the revelation that some people routinely lick the platen clean, for example pupils and dinner supervisors routinely licking their fingers and then rubbing the platen to polish it. By no stretch of the imagination can this be seen as representing good practice in ICT use, and it represents a fairly damning indictment of the system's lack of usability if routinely licking the equipment is seen as practical and necessary.

4. Parental surveillance

A significant number of pupils had experienced problems with parents inspecting digital records of what they had purchased in the cafeteria. For example, one child had dropped her lunch by accident and been forced to purchase a second meal. Her mother had accused her of being greedy and eating two lunches. Several children reported incidences where someone had been bullied by another pupil tipping up their tray as they were carrying it, again either leaving them without lunch or forcing them to buy a second one and having this recorded on the system. Finally one child reported being told off for only having snacks and then skipping lunch. When asked about this, she said, 'My mother "has a little word" with me if I eat jelly and no lunch'.[6]

In this chapter we have explored the implications surrounding the wide-scale collection and storage of children's biometric data in English schools, initially with particular reference to the period between 2006 and 2011. We found that during this period, schools:

1. freely collected biometric data with little concern for children's data privacy rights;

2. had staff and pupils who are persuaded by the convenience of such systems to a point that they do not reflect on the potential social harms, or related legal issues;

3. did not have effective data protection policy or practice in place to be able to manage data such as biometrics effectively and in a legally compliant manner.

By 2015, parental consent compliance had improved, but a number of attitudinal changes had taken place in that some schools had started to get rid of their biometric systems, while others were experiencing significant usability problems relating to pupil resistance, pupil mistrust, hygiene issues, and parental surveillance concerns. This suggests that in the medium to long term, biometric systems may not present the advantages to schools that vendors may originally have indicated. The problems being experienced range from the relatively trivial (licking technological equipment clean), to the more significant (whether enabling a system that indirectly contributes to pupils stealing food has other societal implications).

While we saw no malicious intent around the uncontrolled collection of biometric data, either before or after the 2012 Protection of Freedoms Act, we also observed no reflection on the potential future impacts of such, which suggests that the situation is unresolved and representative of a greater tension, even after nine years. This is the desire to achieve a sophisticated degree of control over young people herded in ever larger groups, at minimal cost, and with little regard to the development of their identities as future citizens in a democratic society. To draw on Baudrillard, we might see this as an example of the 'masses' being trained to be hyper-compliant and unthinking in their response to authority, which in turn sees them in an objectified, commoditized, inauthentic manner. As he argues:

> The masses no longer make themselves evident as a class (a category which has lost its force because of a proliferation of possible identities); they have been swamped by so much meaning that they have lost all meaning. They have been so continuously analysed through statistics, opinion polls and marketing that they do not respond to enlightened political representation.
>
> (Baudrillard, 1983: 19)

Paradoxically, we see that even though children have not finished growing, their bodies are being forced into a model of regulation that assumes a static physical state rather than the dynamic, changing one characteristic of childhood. This in turn raises questions around the role of children in our society – are they equal citizens or some sort of 'other' social group? In the case of the schools in our research, they appear to have been treated as 'other', with their data privacy rights failing to be respected.

Notes

[1] The Panoptic era, in comparison, related to a period in which the design of buildings was meant to enforce self-regulation as the occupants would never know if they were being observed. The term was derived from Bentham's 'Panopticon', a type of prison with a central darkened guard tower surrounded by individual cells that were permanently lit. A detailed description and analysis can be accessed at www.ucl.ac.uk/Bentham-Project/who/panopticon (UCL, 2015).

[2] www.openrightsgroup.org/ (accessed 5 July 2016).

[3] www.no2id.net/ (accessed 5 July 2016).

[4] www.leavethemkidsalone.com (accessed July 30 2012); archived at http://web.archive.org/web/20130401191453/http://www.leavethemkidsalone.com/ (accessed 5 July 2016).

[5] This is a national database containing 5,500 schools across the UK that have been involved in a large-scale e-Safety school self-review process over a period of five years. See Phippen (2014).

[6] This represented one incidence where it must be recorded that the research team, who are parents themselves, clearly and obviously sympathized with the mother's intentions during the focus group.

Chapter 4

Being safe online: The UK education system and safeguarding

There was a time when pushing teenage boundaries at school meant having a quick cigarette with friends behind the school bicycle shed, a light-hearted rite of passage many experienced and which was soon forgotten. Peter Woods includes an example of this in a chapter on 'Having a laugh', in his seminal ethnography of a secondary school, representing it as relatively harmless, and describing it as 'The Smoking Game'. In his book, there is an example of typical teenage smoking banter:

> 'Give us a fag, scruff.'
> 'I don't smoke.'
> 'What are these, then?' (*Fumbling in his pockets*)
> 'Do you want a light?'
>
> (Woods, 1979: 112–4)

For twenty-first-century children, the stakes have become much higher, and there is rarely a time when they are not on public display, whether that is when posting in a computer forum, under CCTV surveillance, being filmed on smartphones, or communicating with others via social media posts that have the capability of being archived in the long term. To use a dramaturgical metaphor from Goffman (1959), for the current generation, there is no longer much backstage space for them to occupy. Their identities are formed and played out almost entirely in the public domain, and this includes at school.

This shift in the nature of privacy brings its own risks. It has also engendered a state of continual anxiety amongst many adults as they seek to protect the young from a threat they may not fully understand or be able to define. In this sense, the ubiquitous nature of contemporary technology means that the role of adults in relation to children is being revisited daily, and with it the very nature of childhood itself is continually changing. Throughout this book we have explored a number of issues related to the way technology has the potential to erode particular aspects of childhood, in particular issues related to the abuse of data, the practice of excessive data collection and sharing, and the increased use of technology by schools to monitor young people's attendance, performance, and even food consumption. We have also argued that, in the absence of effective debate around such issues, we are failing young people. They are increasingly turning to their peers in order to develop knowledge of the adult world, even when this is taking place in the public domain, making it potentially fraught with risk. While growing up has always involved a degree of peer-to-peer information transmission, in the past (as in the case of the cigarette behind the bicycle sheds), this was largely transient. Now, such interactions have much more serious consequences as they have the ability to follow young people for the rest of their lives in unwelcome ways.

In the light of these changes, we use this chapter to explore in more depth how technology can affect the social lives of children. We believe that one major fault line here is the inherent weakness of many education systems to engage fully with the more complex aspects of data protection and safeguarding. This needs to be done from policy, practice, and pedagogic perspectives, and proper consideration needs to be given to what any implications might be for child development in a digital age. Digital safeguarding in a hyper-connected, unregulated childhood is anything but a simple process.

In this chapter, we use a case study approach to highlight some of the social problems concerned, drawing on the 360 Degree Safe[1] tool and database. This tool, which is freely available to all schools in the UK, provides schools with the facilities to self-review the policy and practice around online safety and to develop school improvement strategies in order to enhance their own performance in this area. While some of the scope of the tool falls outside the discussions in this book, the database does provide a number of measures around issues such as data protection, the technical security of data, and the training of staff and governors, all of which contribute to a broad picture of the capabilities of schools to manage (or indeed mismanage) the increasingly complex levels of data they collect and store around pupils in their care. The database paints a consistent picture of schools implementing policy and technical countermeasures to protect children with due diligence, but throws into sharp relief the failure of many schools to a manage risks properly.

There is some hope on the horizon. The impact of school inspection on the motivation of schools to engage with online safety is reassuring, which in the UK is showing shifts in school practice following changes to the Ofsted inspection regime (Ofsted, 2014; 2015a). Yet it is clear that as a society, we lack confidence in most of our education systems when it comes to collecting and managing children's data. Without effective legislative or regulatory change, the status quo will be maintained, and improvement will be slow. However, even with such change, the question of how to find a balance around the issue of children's data rights will always be fraught.

Are schools safeguarding children and their data effectively?

We move now to examine the situation of the UK in more detail. In exploring issues related to children's safeguarding and digital technology, one might ask, 'So what? Why is it important that schools are safeguarding children and their data effectively?' We think there are a number of reasons why this is important, with two being particularly significant:

1. The increased volume of data collected by young people presents significant data protection risks. We see a growing use of biometrics in schools and the routine collection of large quantities of data for all manner of reasons, such as attendance, reading habits, lunchtime consumption, behaviour, homework, and attainment. Increasingly multiple stakeholders are able to access this data (for example, parents, senior leaders, or governors). The UK presents an extreme example of this situation, as discussed in Chapter 6.

2. With the post-2010 increase in the number of academies, a kind of autonomous school free to commission its own technology provision, we have seen an increase in the number of cloud-based providers for such systems. This adds another level of complexity to data protection issues. It is particularly the case in the event that the physical storage of data in these systems resides outside the EU – for example, in the US – and therefore not legislated under EU General Data Protection Directives (European Union, 2016). These jurisdictional boundaries have been the focus of much data protection discussion since the European Courts of Justice ruling on the unenforceable nature of the Safe Harbour agreement[2] on the EU Data Protection Directive,[3] such that data stored in the US on EU citizens would not be bound by this legislation. Therefore, third parties that may have interests in the data collected in UK schools for commercial purposes may even have claim to such data if a school has not paid sufficient due diligence to where it is stored. In such a case, the pupils of the school essentially become a

potential product to be pushed towards advertisers, even though their parents may not have consented to this explicitly.

Much of the data collected is innocuous when taken in isolation. However when aggregated it can become extremely valuable. For example, produce companies may wish to look for particular regions where certain types of food are popular, behaviour management system providers may be interested if a school has an issue with discipline, or education service providers may wish to target the parents of low-achieving pupils to offer support or tutoring services. Without awareness of data protection responsibilities, effective technical infrastructure, and lack of staff and governor training, all of this data may be placed at risk and potentially impact on young people's privacy, development, and future lives.

This is already starting to occur. We regularly see examples of cloud-based data breaches when carrying out research fieldwork. In one case, we were observing an educational institution where a US-based cloud server was used to collect the CVs of students as part of a careers development exercise, with all students being granted access to the folder used. This single scenario creates great potential for the uncontrolled collection of personal data from the students. When the teachers concerned were challenged about this, their response was that it surely could not be 'too bad' if someone obtained the CV of a fellow student. Possibly not, but such matters need to be given fuller consideration if schools are to stay the right side of the law, let alone any kind of professional moral code.

As schools and universities continue to collect increasing volumes of data on their pupils, we raise the issue of whether institutions are aware and knowledgeable enough to ensure that such data is collected in a responsible and safe way, and that this is not open to abuse. There is another more existential issue that arises as our young people are increasingly measured, monitored, and tracked. They are passive in this process, receiving little education around social issues such as respect, consent, boundaries, rights, and risk related to the impact of digital technology on their lives. Consequently there is a serious risk that the next generation of our society develops in a way that makes them think they have no right to privacy. Young people will be growing up with multiple forms of technological intervention, data collection, and monitoring, without effective protection and education, and this is becoming normalized. As we discuss in Chapter 5, the redistribution of explicit images of peers is viewed, by some, to be mundane or even tiresome, and certainly not something worthy of challenge. If we compound a perception of the lack of a right to privacy in their social lives with a view that it is perfectly acceptable to be fingerprinted at school, to post their CV up for public consumption to a large-scale forum, to have their internet access monitored and challenged, and to be presented with their school life plotted as points on a kind of educational 'flight path', we can see a worrying ideology completely at odds with the UN 'Convention on the rights of the child' (UN General Assembly, 1990), in particular Article 16:

> **Article 16 (Right to privacy)**: Children have a right to privacy. The law should protect them from attacks against their way of life, their good name, their families and their homes.

And also Article 29:

> **Article 29 (Goals of education)**: Children's education should develop each child's personality, talents and abilities to the fullest. It should encourage children to respect others, human rights and their own and other cultures. It should also help them learn to live peacefully, protect the environment and respect other people…

Therefore, in this chapter we focus on evaluating schools' effectiveness at addressing these issues. We examine how they ensure data is collected in a secure, responsible, and appropriate manner, whether the importance of security and privacy is understood by those in control of data, and whether young people receive relevant and up-to-date education about their digital rights. Prior to exploring the evidence base in depth, we reflect on the current state of the schools inspectorate in England, given their influence on school policy and practice, as a potential driver for change in UK schools.

The role of the schools inspectorate as a driver for change

The Office for Standards in Education, Children's Services and Skills (Ofsted) is the schools inspectorate for state-funded schools in England. Its role is to:[4]

> …inspect and regulate services that care for children and young people, and services providing education and skills for learners of all ages…

As part of the scrutiny on schools practice and governance, Ofsted plays a major part in making public judgements that are published on its website. In that way, it is an extremely powerful influencer of senior leaders in schools, as a poor Ofsted inspection can result in the replacing of management and governance in a school.

This has been compounded by the Academies Act 2010 (UK Government, 2010), which enabled the 'academization' of all state schools so that they could be decoupled from local authority control and funded directly from the Department for Education. A further aim of the act was to place greater autonomy in the hands of school leaders and governing bodies in matters such as staff salaries and curriculum diversity. Arguably, in decoupling schools from local authority control, Ofsted now provides the only challenge to the senior management of any academy school outside local governance. Prior to the academization programme, schools were funded through the local authority, which provided scrutiny of school practice, school improvement staff, and objective support and challenge to schools. Without local authority influence, school governance became in essence the school senior leadership and the board of governors at the school. The board would generally comprise unpaid volunteers[5] from the local population (for example, parent governors whose children are at the school) and the wider business community (particularly given the advent of private sector investment in academies) who are in place to provide challenge to the senior team and make decisions related to school strategy and governance. Therefore, if effective steering is not provided via the governing body, the only other challenge to the senior team at a school, outside of legislation, is arguably the inspectorate itself.

The inspectorate therefore has a great deal of influence over the priorities set in schools by leaders: if schools are aware they will be inspected on a specific aspect of education policy or practice, they are more likely to invest time and effort in it. As such, when the inspectorate explicitly defines an interest in a particular area, or sets a precedent through an inspection, it can have a significant influence on practice in schools.

In September 2012 Ofsted released a report on 'Inspecting safeguarding' (Ofsted, 2012), which referred to 'online safety issues' for the first time:

> Safeguarding is not just about protecting children from deliberate harm. It includes issues for schools such as: ... bullying, including cyber-bullying (by text message, on social networking sites, and so on) ... internet or e-safety...

Paragraph 51:

> ...Inspectors should include e-safety in their discussions with pupils (covering topics such as safe use of the internet and social networking sites, cyber-bullying, including by text message and so on), and what measures the school takes to promote safe use and combat unsafe use, both proactively (by preparing pupils to engage in e-systems) and reactively (by helping them to deal with a situation when something goes wrong).
>
> *(ibid.)*

While this guidance may be interpreted as being purely about the education around being 'safe online', the interpretation of the framework was evidenced to encapsulate safeguarding around data management and access control in an inspection of a school in 2013, which was specifically critical of school leadership due to failures in authentication, auditability, and the management of internet access at the school:

> Leadership and management are inadequate and behaviour and safety requires improvement because school leaders have failed to ensure that access to the school site and to all parts of the school's computer systems are secure.
>
> Ensure, as a matter of urgency, that:
>
> • an external review of site security is carried out and school leaders respond rapidly and in full to its findings
> • the school follows its policy to ensure that all students and adults accessing computer systems have a unique and secure username and password so that internet access and use can be monitored
>
> (Ofsted, 2013)

In a further indication of a commitment to inspect such issues explicitly, the 2015 Ofsted Common Inspection Framework (Ofsted, 2015b) went into more detail on digital issues, particularly in relation to safeguarding:

> 10. Safeguarding action may be needed to protect children and learners from ... bullying, including online bullying and prejudice-based bullying ... the impact of new technologies on sexual behaviour, for example sexting...

11. Safeguarding is not just about protecting children, learners and vulnerable adults from deliberate harm, neglect and failure to act. It relates to broader aspects of care and education, including ... online safety and associated issues ... Inspectors should include online safety in their discussions with pupils and learners (covering topics such as online bullying and safe use of the internet and social media). Inspectors should investigate what the school or further education and skills provider does to educate pupils in online safety and how the provider or school deals with issues when they arise.

(*ibid.*)

Within this document the inspectorate also defined what they understood by the term 'online safety':

The term 'online safety' reflects a widening range of issues associated with technology and a user's access to content, contact with others and behavioural issues.

(*ibid.*)

This is a far broader and more inclusive definition that those defined in recent years by policymakers, whose focus seems more on prevention of access to inappropriate content (for example, see Baroness Howe's Online Safety Bill being debated in the House of Lords at the time of writing) (UK Government, 2016) rather than looking at a broad range of education and safeguarding issues.

In this review, we can see that with increased attention from the inspectorate, there is certainly external pressure on senior leaders to engage with the issues around online safety – on which, given the inspectorate's own definition, we would place the focus of discussion in this text. We will explore the impact of changes in inspection as we explore the 360 Degree Safe database.

The 360 Degree Safe tool and its role in measuring school policy, practice, and education provision

The 360 Degree Safe tool was developed by the South West Grid for Learning (SWGfL),[6] a not-for-profit Internet Service Provider (ISP) and internet advisory service used by the majority of schools in the South West of England. SWGfL draws upon the experience of leading practitioners in the field, all of whom have had considerable experience in the field of online safety, whether as school leaders, teachers, academics, or technology specialists. The trust was originally funded by 15 local authorities, as described in Phippen (2013), but since the distancing of local authorities from education funding as a result of the Academies Act (*ibid.*), the charity now generates its own funding through interactions with schools and the wider children's workforce. The tool was originally launched as a paper-based system in November 2009, after first being piloted in the South West region. It was then refined and launched as a web-based tool. Since its launch, it has won a number of national awards and is widely recognized, including by the schools inspectorate Ofsted, as the de facto standard for online safety review in the UK, and is currently in use, voluntarily, by almost a third of schools across the country.

Content and structures of the 360 Degree Safe tool

Schools carry out e-safety self-reviews via a web interface, and the data are sent to a centralized relational database. This database holds the information in three related tables, categorized as Establishments, Aspects, and Rating. The schools complete each 'aspect' against which they self-review their level, which is stored as a rating in the database. Each aspect can be rated between level 5, the weakest, and level 1, the strongest, depending on where the school's own practice sits:

Table 4.1: 360 Degree Safe levels

Level 5	There is little or nothing in place
Level 4	Policy and practice is being developed
Level 3	Basic e-safety policy and practice is in place
Level 2	Policy and practice is coherent and embedded
Level 1	Policy and practice is aspirational and innovative

For each aspect in the tool, there is clear guidance and definition for each level, as well as guidance on how to progress to the next level of each aspect – hence the tool can be used for school improvement as well as baseline measurement. Schools are able to log in and upgrade their scores when they feel they have reached a new level, so the database holds a record of their progress, as well as their baseline. In order to illustrate the level of detail, the levels for the personal data aspect are defined in Table 4.2:

Table 4.2: Data protection aspect levels

Data Protection
This aspect describes the ability of the school to be compliant with Data Protection and Freedom of Information legislation. It describes the ability of the school to effectively control practice through the implementation of policy, procedure, and education of all users.

Level 5	There are no policies ensuring compliance with legal, statutory, regulatory, and contractual data requirements. The school has not yet registered with the ICO.
Level 4	The school is developing a comprehensive Data Protection Policy. The school has registered with the ICO. Parents and carers are informed about their rights and about the use of personal data through the Privacy Notice.
Level 3	The school has a comprehensive Data Protection Policy. All staff know and understand their statutory obligations under the Data Protection Act to ensure the safe keeping of personal data, minimizing the risk of its loss or misuse. Parents and carers are informed about their rights and about the use of personal data through the Privacy Notice. The school has processes in place to manage Freedom of Information requests. The governors/directors are involved in the development and approval of Data Protection Policy and control processes. The school has undertaken an audit to identify the personal and sensitive data it processes. Personal data is only stored in the cloud where appropriate and measures are in place to secure it which meet with statutory requirements.
Level 2	The school has a comprehensive Data Protection Policy which addresses issues such as (but not limited to) the use of personal devices and those devices that move between school and beyond; cloud storage; personal data; monitoring, device management, and asset tracking; filtering, firewall rules, passwords, and disposal. These policies are known, understood, and adhered to by users. Parents and carers are informed about their rights and about the use of personal data through the Privacy Notice. The school has processes in place to manage Freedom of Information requests. The governing body is aware of its obligations under the Data Protection Act. Resources are allocated to Data Protection, which is standing agenda

	item. The school has undertaken an audit to identify the personal and sensitive data it processes. Personal data is only stored in the cloud where appropriate and measures are in place to secure it which meet with statutory requirements. Data protection is enhanced through the use of encryption/two-factor authentication for the handling or transfer of sensitive data. The organization has appointed a Data Protection Officer (internally or externally) and Information Asset Owners.
Level 1	The school has a comprehensive Data Protection Policy which addresses issues such as (but not limited to) the use of personal devices and those devices that move between school and beyond; cloud storage; personal data; monitoring, device management, and asset tracking; filtering, firewall rules, passwords, and disposal. The policies make provision for the school to support staff/governors/pupils/students who may access school systems from beyond the school. These policies are known, understood, and adhered to by users. Parents and carers are informed about their rights and about the use of personal data through the Privacy Notice. The school has processes in place to manage Freedom of Information requests. There is an appointed Data Protection Governor and the governing body is aware of its obligations under the Data Protection Act. Resources are allocated to Data Protection, which is standing agenda item. The school has undertaken an audit to identify the personal and sensitive data it processes. Personal data is only stored in the cloud where appropriate and measures are in place to secure it which meet with statutory requirements. Data protection is enhanced through the use of encryption/two-factor authentication for the handling or transfer of sensitive data. The organization has appointed a Data Protection Officer (internally or externally) and Information Asset Owners. All protected data is clearly labelled. There is a clear procedure in place for audit logs to be kept and for reporting, managing, and recovering from information risk incidents.

In total, there are 28 aspects defined in the tool, grouped first by 'elements' (overarching themes in school governance), 'strands' (logical groupings of aspects within elements, for example, policies), and then the individual 'aspects' themselves:

Table 4.3: 360 Degree Safe structure

Elements	Strands	Aspects
Policy and leadership	Responsibilities	E-safety group E-safety responsibilities Governors
	Policies	Policy development Policy scope Acceptable use agreement Self-evaluation Whole school Sanctions Reporting
	Communications and communication technologies	Mobile devices Social media Digital and video images Public online communications Professional standards
Infrastructure	Passwords	Password security
	Services	Connectivity and filtering Technical security Personal data
Education	Children and young people	E-safety education Digital literacy The contribution of young people
	Staff	Staff training
	Governors	Governor training
	Parents and carers	Parental education
	Community	Community engagement
Standards and inspection	Monitoring	Impact of e-safety policy and practice
		Monitoring the impact of the e-safety policy and practice

Validity of school self-review data

The question of whether schools can be relied upon to self-report their compliance situation accurately needs to be raised. School self-review is now considered a mainstream activity in many countries, particularly the UK (Shewbridge *et al.*, 2014) and New Zealand (Nusche *et al.*, 2012), where the Organization for Economic Co-operation and Development (OECD) has recently sponsored evaluation activities demonstrating success. For some time, however, school self-review processes were seen as being potentially prone to bias and inconsistency. In its early days, Pring (1996) and Elliott (1996) argued against relying on school self-review data as a vehicle for school improvement. However MacBeath (1999), Barber (1997), Mortimore and Sammons (1997), Mortimore and Whitty (1997), and Stoll (1992) all provide counterarguments disputing any lack of reliability and validity. School self-review was thought by these authors to allow unique insight into many aspects of education and school life that eluded formal inspection. This certainly would appear to have been the case in relation to the 360 Degree Safe tool, as it tracks attitudes towards online safety, something that is difficult to record using alternative mechanisms. We can also argue that, for an area such as online safety, what is the benefit in overinflated measures? This is not a metric used by inspectors to assess performance, although schools have used carrying the e-Safety Mark (see below) as evidence of good practice to inspectors, it merely provides the means for a school to determine their own fit. While 360 Degree Safe has been used by Ofsted to discuss online safety (Ofsted, 2015c), inspectors will still ask questions around online safety practice and policy: they will not blithely follow the metrics in the tool. Finally, as the tool's use continues to become more widespread, with increasing numbers of schools involved, reliability is also increasing. The database is analysed every year and has resulted in annual 'state of the nation' reports published by the SWGfL (for example, see Phippen, 2010; 2012a; 2013). In each of these cases, while there is overall improvement against aspects, the 'shape' of the data has remained consistent, even with the addition of new establishments every year. This would indicate a strength of validity of the data since the early adopters certainly did not present a different overall profile to those who are just starting to use the tool now.

As the practice of school self-review has become more established and nuanced over the years, Kyriakides and Campbell (2004) and Schildkampa *et al.* (2009) have argued that a strong set of evaluation criteria is the key to ensuring success and reliability. In the case of the 360 Degree Safe tool, a highly structured approach, underpinned with extremely clear definitions and guidance, is used. This suggests that the data are likely to be sufficiently reliable for our purposes, namely the assessment and changing of teachers' and school administrators' attitudes towards online safety.

By way of a final validity measure, the SWGfL also provides an accreditation process for schools wishing to gain external recognition for their online safety policy and practice – the 'e-Safety Mark'.[7] The provision of an inspection visit for schools that wish to apply for accreditation in online safety serves to enhance reliability and validity. While it has to be noted that schools self-select for accreditation and are therefore more likely to have achieved maturity in their compliance processes, such inspection visits during the life of the project (120 to date) have confirmed school self-review data in each case, indicating that schools were generally accurate in their self-assessments about their online safety practices.

Analysis of the 360 Degree Safe dataset

Analysis of the data focuses on establishment's self-review of their online safety policy and practice, exploring their ratings against the 28 aspects of 360 Degree Safe. However, for the sake of the analysis in this text, we will not be exploring the full aspects set. Given our focus on data and privacy abuses, alongside ineffective education around social aspects of living in a hyper-connected society, we will draw on the data from 15 different aspects that cover the main areas that feature in Department for Education guidance (DfE, 2016 this reference is missing) and ICO guidance (ICO, 2007), as well as those aspects that underpin the education offer in schools. Again, drawing from the definitions in the 360 Degree Safe tool, these are:

Acceptable use agreement: how a school communicates its expectations for acceptable use of technology and the steps towards successfully implementing them in a school. This is supported by evidence of users' awareness of their responsibilities.

Connectivity and filtering: a school's ability to manage access to content across its systems and monitor activity to safeguard users. This includes filtering technologies, network monitoring, and reporting and incident management.

E-Safety education: how the school builds resilience in its pupils/students through an effective online safety education programme.

E-Safety responsibilities: the roles of those responsible for the school's online safety strategy.

Governors: governors' safety accountability and how the school ensures this influences policy and practice.

Governor training: the school's provision for the online safety education of governors to support them in the execution of their role.

Password security: the ability of the school to ensure the security of its systems and data through good password policy and practice. It addresses the need for age-appropriate password practices, and for the school to implement password records, recovery, and change routines.

Personal data: the ability of the school to comply with Data Protection and Freedom of Information legislation. It describes the ability of the school to control practice effectively through the implementation of policy, procedure, and education of all users.

Policy development: the process of establishing an effective online safety policy: the stakeholders involved and their responsibilities, which are: consultation, communication, review, and impact.

Policy scope: policy content; its breadth in terms of technology and expectations around behaviour and its relevance to current social trends and educational developments.

Public online communications: how the school manages its public-facing online communications, both in managing risk and disseminating online safety advice, information, and practice.

Reporting: the routes and mechanisms the school provides for its community to report abuse and misuse.

Sanctions: the actions a school may take and the strategies it employs in response to misuse. There is evidence that responsible use is acknowledged through celebration and reward.

Staff training: the effectiveness of the school's online safety staff development programme and how it prepares and empowers staff to educate and intervene in issues when they arise.

Technical security: the ability of the school to understand and ensure reasonable duty of care regarding the technical and physical security of administrative and curriculum networks (including Wi-Fi) and devices and the safety of its users.

The 360 Degree Safe tool is 'live', so it is not possible to draw a conclusive dataset: the data are constantly evolving as establishments embark on their self-review or continue with school improvements around online safety. Therefore, in order to analyse the dataset, it is necessary to take a data snapshot on a given date. For the purposes of this analysis the data snapshot was taken on 30 September 2015. In total from this capture there are almost 7,000 registrations logged (representing approximately 35 per cent of schools in the UK):

Table 4.4: Overall registrations for the SWGfL tool

Establishments signed up to the tool at 30 September 2015	6950
Establishments that have embarked on the self-review process	4507
Establishments with full profiles completed	2834

Of these establishments, we had a broad geographical spread:

Table 4.5: Registrations by region for the SWGfL tool

Channel Islands	29
London	623
Midlands	1497
North East	597
North West	848
Overseas	18
South East	1187
South West	1816

The overseas establishments that are registered generally comprise service schools abroad that are still considered part of the UK educational establishment profile, such as services schools overseas. A number of establishments had not specified a location, which is why that total does not add up to the full 6,950. However, we are not measuring on region but the dataset as a whole, to use this metric as an index of the geographical spread of establishments. We can see there is broad engagement across the country as a whole, and not only the South West.

As a final demographic measure, we can determine the number of schools per phase, which is detailed in Table 4.6. The majority of establishments are in either a primary or secondary setting, with a higher proportion of those being primaries (which we would expect given the higher proportion of primary schools in the education setting). The 'not applicable' establishments are such entities as special schools, local authorities, and informal education providers.

Table 4.6: Phase of registrants for the SWGfL tool

All through	25
Not applicable	154
Nursery	39
Primary	4590
Secondary	2142

Overall performance measures

Statistics are measured based on the best rating any given establishment has posted for each aspect, therefore giving the strongest and most up-to-date performances by establishments. If we consider the mean values per aspect in the dataset, we can see stronger and weaker performing areas in schools, as illustrated in Figure 4.1. Note that '5' is the weakest value and '1' the strongest, so the lower the value the better the performance:

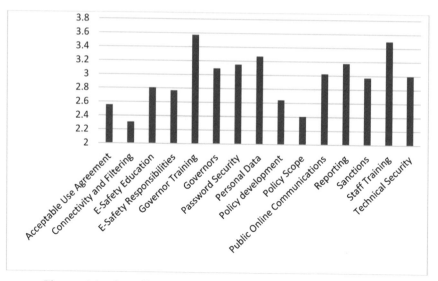

Figure 4.1: Overall mean values per aspect across the whole SWGfL dataset

From this data, we can see that areas of strength lie predominantly in the policy and technical areas. The strongest aspects are:

- Connectivity and filtering (2.309)
- Policy scope (2.406)
- Acceptable use agreement (2.554)

- Policy development (2.642)
- E-Safety responsibilities (2.767)

We can therefore see that policies in the online safety areas are generally at least in place (bearing in mind that level 3 is a basic level of policy or practice), and 'connectivity and filtering' are strong, being closer to good practice on average. This is not surprising given that this is a capital investment, usually provided off the shelf by a third party, and requires little resource commitment other that maintenance.

However, if we consider the weakest aspects in more detail, we see a worrying trend:

- Governor training (3.574)
- Staff training (3.498)
- Personal data (3.27)
- Reporting (3.175)
- Password security (3.151)

From the weakest aspects within our subset of aspects focusing more on the data protection area, we can note with some concern that 'password security' is one of the weakest areas, given that this aspect explores how effectively schools implement access control on the school systems. However, perhaps even more concerning is that the two weakest aspects are those upon which a school would be most reliant in understanding the nature of data protection and safeguarding within the school setting. If both staff and governor knowledge are poor (and in both cases averages are below 'basic' practice, indicating that a large number of establishments do not have either in place) there is little likelihood that the complex issues around data protection or safeguarding are well understood, and an effective challenge to senior management on these matters certainly cannot exist.

If we consider the standard deviations of the whole dataset, we see a range of breadths of distribution, which hold different meanings for different aspects.

For example, given that 'connectivity and filtering' is the strongest aspect and the narrowest standard deviation, we can be confident that this aspect is strong across the majority of schools in our dataset. However, for weaker aspects such as 'personal data' and 'staff training', having a narrow distribution is a negative measure. Given the importance of a measure such as 'personal data', which helps us to understand whether schools have a policy in place to ensure they are managing students' personal data effectively and responsibly, it is not reassuring to see that we have a low mean and narrow standard deviation, given that this implies the majority of schools have weak practice in this area. Having an even narrower standard deviation for 'staff training' again increases our concerns about the existing level of knowledge regarding data protection and safeguarding.

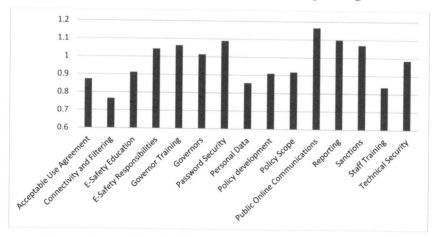

Figure 4.2: Overall standard deviations per aspect of the SWGfL dataset

A further analysis of the distribution of ratings can be seen if we look at the spread of each aspect per level and consider how many schools have rated themselves as level 1, level 2, etc. This is illustrated in Figure 4.3:

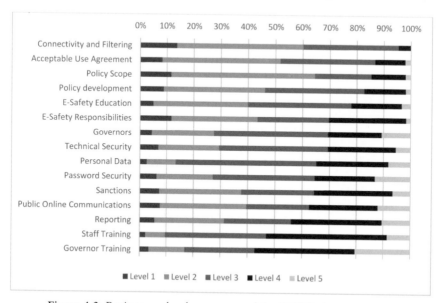

Figure 4.3: Ratings per level per aspect of the SWGfL dataset

We have ranked these based upon the proportion of schools that have rated themselves between level 1 and 3 (meaning they have at least some policy or practice in place) in an aspect. From this ranking we can see, again, that connectivity and policy areas are generally very strong, with the vast majority of schools having at least basic provision in place. We may, however, still raise concerns that around 15 per cent of schools in the dataset have no 'acceptable usage agreement' in place, which means subsequent response to breaches, abuse on systems, or unauthorized access, has no underpinning policy support and therefore legislative protection.

If we look at personal data, which is mid-ranking in terms of overall performance, we can see that by far the most common rating for this aspect is a level 3, denoting basic implementation of a data protection policy that adheres to legislation set out under the Data Protection Act. However, once again the main concern obviously arises with the weakly performing areas, particularly around training, given we can see that in terms of both staff and governors, around 50 per cent of schools have no training in place at all. Furthermore, the weakness of the reporting aspect is worrying, with almost 50 per cent of schools having no established reporting routes for abuse and misuse. This would suggest that, in the event of a data breach or report of, for example, online harassment, the school has no mechanism in place for responding to the situation and will therefore be reactive, rather than proactive.

In exploring the data in more detail, a useful decomposition to clarify our understanding of schools' performance across our dataset further is to separate out primary and secondary schools. A top-level analysis of this is presented in Figure 4.4, which presents the mean values per aspect of primary and secondary establishments.

From this analysis we can see that, in general, primary schools will underperform secondaries. On one level this is unsurprising, given the resourcing implications of some of these aspects. One would expect a secondary school, with generally larger budgets and staffing, to be able to be stronger in these areas. However, there is a less clear explanation for some of the policy-focused aspects, given that these are less resource intensive. We can see, for example, that personal data is a far weaker aspect in primary schools. Given the 360 Degree Safe tool will go as far as providing template policies, it is unclear why primaries are so much weaker, unless it results from school governance simply not acknowledging this area as important to the setting. Furthermore, while there are some areas where there is greater strength in primary schools, for example in aspects related to governors, the differences are not as great for those where they are weaker.

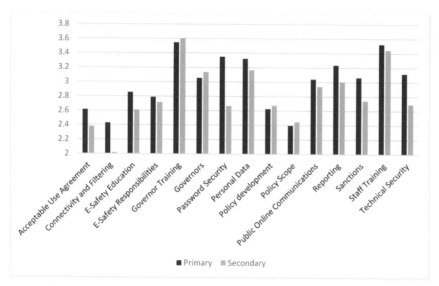

Figure 4.4: Comparison of primary and secondary averages in the SWGfL dataset

The distribution of the weakest areas for primary and secondary schools are illustrated in figures 4.5 and 4.6:

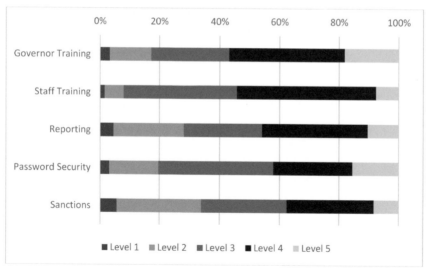

Figure 4.5: Weakest aspects for primary schools based on distribution in the SWGfL dataset

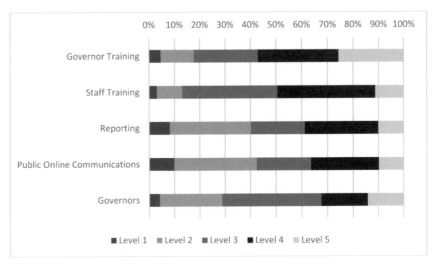

Figure 4.6: Weakest aspects in secondary schools based on distribution in the SWGfL dataset

We can see from these two graphs that the three weakest aspects – 'governor training', staff training', and 'reporting' – generally have parity across the two settings, though more secondary schools than primaries have a good level of reporting in place. However, the variations between the two settings with the other two weakest aspects are interesting. For primary schools we see greater weakness in 'password security' (ensuring effective access control across the school) and 'sanction' (being able to deal with the aftermath of digitally related incidents in a well thought-out structured manner). When dealing with data, and looking after the sensitive data related to young children, this is very much a concern. In the secondary settings, there is weakness in terms of articulating to the wider school community issues related to staying safe online, protecting personal data, and similar concerns. We also see that almost 40 per cent of secondary schools have no clearly defined roles and responsibilities for governors in this area.

Finally, given the focus in this chapter on the importance of schools, which collect increasing amounts of data on their pupils for all manner of reasons, to have effective data protection measures and compliance in place, it is worthwhile comparing the performance of the 'personal data' aspect in each setting.

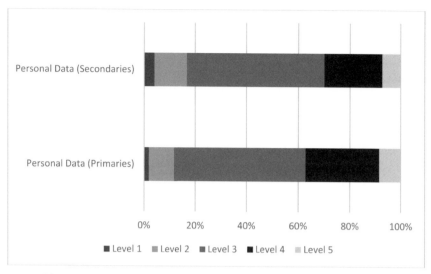

Figure 4.7: Comparison of data protection aspects of the SWGfL dataset

From this we can see that by far the most common level is 3, which denotes basic practice (and is defined in more detail in Table 4.1). However, more worrying is that almost 40 per cent of primary schools, and over 30 per cent of secondaries, have no policy in place around this aspect. This aspect is fundamental to any understanding and implementation of data protection, and defining proper roles and responsibilities is absolutely key here. If we look back at the earlier discussion in this chapter around the capabilities of schools in the UK to manage the increasing level of personal data pertaining to pupils across numerous systems, it is hard to have confidence in school policies if this responsibility has not been properly met.

All these analyses raise the question of how a school can improve its approach to data protection and the safeguarding of digital issues. As discussed above, the schools' inspectorate has specifically stated since September 2012 that online safety issues will be part of both safeguarding and general inspections. Through analysis of the dataset we can show the impact of this change in inspection approach. In Figure 4.8, we show raw activity on the tool per month: that is, the volume in a given month of either new ratings being posted or updates to the ratings of established aspects. We can see the typical school cycle in the results, with greater activity in term times and a drop-off during holiday times. We can also see that there has been a general increase in the volume of transactions as more schools have started to use the tool. Since September 2012 in particular, we can see a clear increase in activity with the tool.

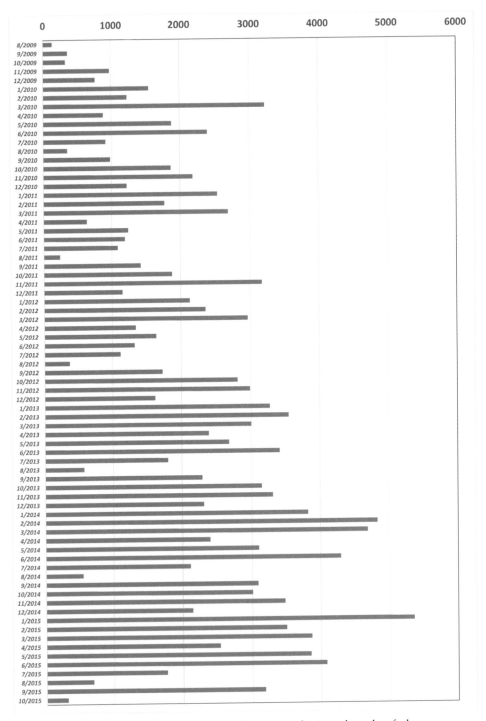

Figure 4.8: Activity on the tool per month since launch of the SWGfL tool

In order to determine whether policy change has resulted in an increase in activity, we can look at activity per year against the total number of ratings posted. The addition of new institutions has led to increased activity post-September 2012. This is associated with steady growth in the use of the tool generally. While we cannot prove that this increase in activity is a result of greater attention from Ofsted, we can certainly show more activity since the changes in inspection framework.

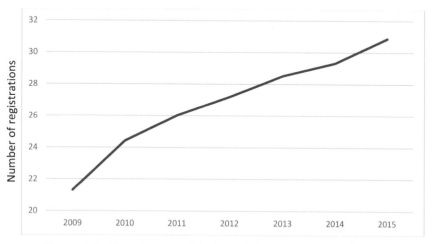

Figure 4.9: Cumulative activity/cumulative registrations for the SWGfL tool

Implications

We can see a number of reasons for schools to increase their collection of data related to their pupils. It is undoubtedly a consequence of the growth of an 'audit culture' within society (Power, 1997; Strathern, 2000; Apple, 2010), where so much is deemed measurable. However, we have already proposed that in some cases, data collection is a by-product of convenience (for example, biometric systems replacing the burden of having to carry a library or lunch card), where the data controllers reflect little on the implications of this increase in collection or the need for protection of this clearly sensitive data.

As we will discuss in Chapter 6, we also see the promotion of these systems as a means of solving other problems faced by school, such as behaviour or safeguarding. Again there is little advice or guidance about how this data should be managed or safeguarded. Nevertheless, what is clear is that this increase in data collection should place a high expectation on those in charge of governance at a school to show responsibility regarding the management of that data, and compliance with the appropriate legislation put in place to ensure effective safeguards are in place.

Yet the protection of personal data, the appropriate technical infrastructure, the incident response mechanisms, and the relevant training of stakeholders have all been shown to be wanting with analysis of data from the 360 Degree Safe tool. Perhaps the most concerning of these is the lack of training of both staff and those who are expected to hold them to account in their data protection and safeguarding responsibilities. Without having the requisite knowledge in the school – and our data has shown that in our sample an extremely high number of schools do not – we cannot expect the subsequent development of effective practice within the establishment, let alone appropriate teaching of data protection issues and management to pupils. The result is therefore education settings where staff are not sufficiently aware of data protection compliance responsibilities. This can place the institution at risk, and staff are also ill-equipped either to deal with behaviours by the pupils in their care or to understand the complexities of their relationship with digital technology, and not sufficiently cognizant of the implications of failing to protect data on the young people in their care effectively. While we have seen that change in policy by the inspectorate can result in changes to governance and practice in schools, with the explicit mention of online safety in Ofsted frameworks from September 2012, we have not seen a subsequent step change. While it has had an impact, this is not culture changing.

In the next chapter, we begin to explore what happens when education settings do not have sufficient policy, mechanisms, and knowledge to deal with the fallout from hyper-connected childhoods through an exploration of the teen sexting phenomenon. However, in contrast to the majority of work in this area, it will not explore the phenomenon itself, but the educational and legislative response to the issues arising from it.

Notes

[1] www.360safe.org.uk (accessed 5 July 2016).
[2] The Safe Harbour agreement was essentially an agreement between EU and US governments to protect EU data when stored in the US.
[3] An ECJ ruling stated that, in the wake of the revelations by Edward Snowden, the Safe Harbour agreement was not legally binding and did not offer legislative data protection of EU citizens' data stored in the US.
[4] www.ofsted.gov.uk (accessed 5 July 2016).
[5] While the changes to school status as a result of the Academies Act does enable provision for school governors to be paid, the vast majority remain unpaid.
[6] www.swgfl.org.uk/ (accessed 5 July 2016).
[7] The e-Safety Mark is an accreditation process conducted by the SWGfL to accredit a school for reaching required levels across the 360 Degree Safe tool. See www.360safe.org.uk/Accreditation/E-Safety-Award (accessed 21 April 2015).

Chapter 5

The new normal? Sexting as a case study of children's risk and stakeholder response

Thinking about the social and biological context of young people's behaviour is important when seeking to understand it, and in this chapter we explore the issue of sexting as well as the school culture surrounding it. We see sexting as another example of what is a kind of analogue behaviour in a digital world, rather like secret smoking as described in Chapter 4. The essence of the behaviour is rooted in the developing sexual identities of adolescents, and has parallels with behaviours in pre-internet society. To give a salacious example, both authors of this book witnessed alarming (and at the time, highly amusing) incidents as pupils on 1980s school trips, mainly involving the back row of the school bus and a choreographed revelation of various parts of the body at unsuspecting car and lorry drivers following behind. Nudity was, and is, considered offensive in the context of schooling, and public exposure in this way has been illegal since Victorian times. Yet this back row behaviour takes place within a liminal space for adolescents, where they are poised between childhood and adulthood – the playfulness of children housed within the developing bodies of youths. Provocative back row behaviour also serves a fundamental and primitive need to bond with the tribe, in social anthropological terms. You are never more included in a group than when you choreograph a mildly illicit act with your peers, and this kind of in-group identification and inclusion is something most adolescents yearn for.

Having established that occasional nudity can play a key role amongst adolescents as a social group, we move now to sexting. The term refers to the self-generation and distribution of explicit images to either one or more recipients. It is a phenomenon of the digital age and consequently attracts much media interest, for example in the *Daily Mail* (2012). The word itself was an Orwellian media creation, a conflation of the sharing of explicit text messages along with self-generated images, a technical capability that became possible in a mainstream context in the early 2000s. An early media focus of sexting was the behaviour of celebrities, when the first high-profile use of the term, which cemented the term in the cultural *zeitgeist*, referred to the Australian cricketer Shane Warne in a report in the Australian *Sunday Telegraph Magazine* (Roberts, 2005). After that, 'sexting' became established in the lexicon of modern technology.

As the phenomenon has taken hold, there has also been a great deal of media interest in young people and sexting, something that is unsurprising given the subject matter and the need to produce stories that result in sales or advertising pay-per-click behaviour. Consequently, the highest profile coverage of teen sexting will be of serious and high-impact incidents. For example, one of the highest profile stories that linked the practice of sexting with adolescent behaviour was the suicide of Jesse Logan (NoBullying, 2015a). In this case Jesse was a teenager who sent her then boyfriend a nude image, which was subsequently distributed by him to others in her school. As a result of this distribution she was severely bullied, which ultimately resulted in her committing suicide. In another case that received high levels of media attention, the Canadian teenager Amanda Todd committed suicide (NoBullying, 2015b) after three years of abuse that had resulted from a sexting-related incident she had carried out with a stranger on a webcam when she was younger.

We take a novel perspective on the role of sexting in the popular culture of young people. In doing so, there are several common themes that this chapter will not cover. Sexting behaviour, attitudes, and culture have all been explored at length and in considerable detail by other authors or in our previous work (for example, Wolak and Finkelhor, 2011; Ringrose *et al.*, 2012; Phippen, 2009), so it will not be the main focus of this chapter. Neither will we try to quantify frequency among young people: again there have been a number of quantitative studies that present such information (for example, A Thin Line, 2011; Phippen, 2009). An additional factor is that realistically, sexting behaviour is a challenging area to measure. Given that the research subjects are aware of the potential legal issues surrounding the practice, it is unlikely a full and frank response will be received from a teenage population, regardless of guarantees of anonymity. We also see little value in presenting another discourse on the practice of sexting as manifested in that demographic, which would surely cover the same points as previous outputs. It is now, nonetheless, well established that sexting goes on, and it is something that schools have to deal with. In a recent talk given by one of the authors to a group of safeguarding leads in the south west of England, when asked if there was anyone present who had never had to deal with a sexting incident in their school, nobody raised a hand. As has been raised in other research (for example, Ringrose *et al.*, 2012; Phippen,

2012b), sexting is 'normal' for many English teenagers: while they may not themselves engage in it, they are aware of it going on and are cognizant of its impact.

This chapter uses sexting as a case study of the failures of education systems to understand fully the issues arising from a digital society, as well as the difficulties of engaging with incidents when they arise. In other words, we discuss the implications of dealing with safeguarding incidents from a position of general ignorance. Schools may be at the front line of digital childhood, but it is becoming increasingly clear that they lack the knowledge base, infrastructure, reporting routes, and governance to address problems adequately. We explore whether the prohibitive ideology that appears to be endemic within most schooling systems will ever successfully prepare children and young people for the reality of the hyper-connected world and its risks. We also explain how falling back on legislative protection and regulation will also be found wanting if the wider context is not fully understood. Finally, we develop the rights perspectives that are a strong theme throughout this book.

At various points within this discussion, this chapter draws on the experiences of the authors working in schools in recent years. These data are generally ethnographic in nature: while there have been occasions when we have visited a school setting with a very specific aim, for example with the discussions around biometrics discussed in Chapter 3, the majority of data is taken from interactions, discussions, and observations within classroom activities and workshops that have no specific research question, but are conducted within a body of work that explores the nature of digital engagement within youth culture, with discussion driven by the young people themselves. We have also been involved in the delivery of many training and awareness sessions to staff members, which allows us to reflect on staff awareness of online safeguarding and protection issues. While this results in unstructured data at a macro level, it does facilitate the exploration of cultural phenomena as they emerge, such as in the case of sexting. It is rare that sexting is the primary focus of a workshop or discussion group in a school setting, however, yet workshop participants will often raise the issue when discussing how digital technology affects their lives. We feel that allowing the concerns of our young research participants to be voiced in this way is crucial if the research field is to move forwards.

So you got naked online?

The above title, taken from a resource by the SWGfL providing schools with support on dealing with sexting incidents (SWGfL, 2015) gets to the crux of the issue within the school setting. While sexting might be the physical vehicle to an incident, in that an image was originally taken by a subject on their mobile phone and then sent to a recipient who might subsequently redistribute this image, the issue is not the act itself but the fact that the image was shared outside the trust boundaries between the original sender and receiver. This represents a breach of privacy to the original sender.

The risk lies in the communication of the image without guarantee of further distribution or deletion. We need to be clear that within the sexting context there are different motivations and acts, for example:

- An image generated by an individual as a result of a request from another;
- An image generated by an individual and sent to a recipient who has not asked for it; and
- An image redistributed by a recipient to further third parties or to a public web archive (for example, a social media page or blog).

Within Chapter 4, we highlighted a number of key risks for schools in delivering their safeguarding responsibilities around digital issues, namely:

- Lack of staff awareness of these issues
- Lack of awareness by those responsible for the strategy and governance of the school and, ultimately, with safeguarding responsibilities
- Lack of reporting mechanisms such that incident response is reactive, rather than proactive
- A lack of effective and relevant education for young people, partly as a result of the first two points above.

Within the phenomenon of sexting, these are all too apparent. In discussions with staff around the topic of sexting, it is not unusual for the first response on being told of the prevalence or awareness of sexting among teenagers to be disbelief or shock. Few schools have any form of incident response, and even fewer pupils, in our experience, are likely to disclose a sexting incident (the main reason being that they do not feel teachers will be understanding or know what to do). On more than one occasion we have been told that sexting is not something the school addresses within the curriculum as they feel coverage of such would encourage their pupils to engage in such practices.

While staff members with safeguarding responsibility are more likely to accept that sexting goes on since they are more likely to have dealt with such incidents, many other staff members are less aware of the phenomenon. Some appear to be extremely resistant to viewing engagement as part of their pastoral duties to their pupils. In one school we worked in, the safeguarding lead developed a schedule of tutorials around the topic for Year 9 students (aged 13–14), and half of the tutors refused to deliver it. This is in stark contrast to discussions with young people, who will usually openly talk about the fact that such practices go on amongst their peer groups, with associated disruptions to friendship and sometimes even abuse. However, perhaps the most worrying common attitude is how mundane it all seems to be to the young people concerned: this is normal to them, and phrases like 'it gets old really quickly', and 'oh yeah, there's normally an image or two flying around' are common. It is interesting to note that perhaps the time when they are most surprised is when talking about a case such as Jesse Logan or Amanda Todd, because many feel that a redistributed image is so run of the mill that they do not appreciate how serious abuse can be as a consequence.

We clearly have a gulf between those living a hyper-connected childhood, and those who are tasked with ensuring their safety and well-being, particularly within the school setting. Without an understanding of the issues associated with sexting or a refusal to engage with such due to what might be perceived as professional risk on the part of the teacher (lessening the chances of a parent being outraged as a result of a child coming home and saying 'sir talked to me about sexting today'), schools and other stakeholders fall back on a prohibitive ideology: 'we must stop them from doing this, so we won't have to address it in school'.

The legality of sexting

The first level of this prohibitive approach is to argue against the legality of the practice, which therefore means that the primary strategy should be one of informing pupils that if they engage in sexting, they are breaking the law. However, while there is legislation that can be applied in sexting cases, it is not always straightforward.

There has been much argument that the main focus on sexting prevention should be around legislation, with both US and European cases of teenagers who had become victims of the further distribution of images of themselves being threatened with prosecution under the relevant legislation related to the making and distribution of indecent images of children (Stone, 2011). With the strict application of the law, this is something that falls under the Protection of Children Act 1978 (UK Government, 1978) in the UK. However, in these cases the sexting phenomenon seems to have been viewed as an entirely new, isolated, practice that has no basis in a broader social context. Specific legislation has therefore been called for to dissuade young people from carrying out such practices in the first place (we frequently see headlines along such lines as 'Sexting could earn teenagers criminal record and a place on sex offenders' register') (Huffington Post, 2014). The belief seems to be that to protect minors from the potential harm that results from such illegal behaviour, threat of prosecution is a more effective approach than remedial or restorative action. These views are certainly not unique to the UK and as noted above, there have been a number of prosecutions in the US for similar behaviours (for example, see Tang, 2012).

However, one might argue that this simplistic approach to a complex social act goes against the intentions of the laws that are now being used (or proposed to be used) to 'scare' minors out of engaging with such practices. Surely, laws such as those prohibiting the manufacturing and distribution of indecent images of minors are there to protect vulnerable children, rather than prosecute them? With the older laws, further complexity resides in the fact that statute was put into place at a time before the phenomenon of self-generation was technologically possible. Certainly in the case of the UK's Protection of Children Act in 1978 (UK Government, 1978) it could not have been foreseen that a scenario might come about where the producer and distributor of the image was also the subject of the image.

In some cases criminal prosecution in the UK appears to conflict with the national Association of Chief Police Officers' advice regarding how the law should intervene on issues of sexting/revenge porn among minors (ACPO, n.d.). The ACPO advice seems to take a more pragmatic view. It argues that a producer in a sexting case, while technically breaking the laws around the distribution of indecent images, is someone who is unlikely to represent a particular threat to anybody in general. Therefore this fails the 'public interest' check[1] when a decision to prosecute is being made by the Crown Prosecution Service (CPS). This particularly applies when it could be argued that the offender is as much a victim as a criminal, a perspective backed up by the CPS (CPS, n.d.). However, both the CPS and ACPO advice does go on to suggest that those who take images from others and redistribute them, and do this repeatedly, should be tackled with the laws that are available to address their behaviour.

It seems that in some of the discussions about the application of laws to these issues all concerned are being viewed as equally guilty of offence and should be treated in the same way. Another particularly troubling aspect of these discussions is that we know it is very unlikely a young person subjected to this sort of abuse would turn to an adult for help. The vast majority of young people in our research said their peers would be the people they would ask. The idea that an adult might help, or even understand, was lost on a lot of young people who felt that if they were to mention such abuse to an adult, they would be 'judged' as having done something wrong (despite statistics that show that almost 50 per cent of adults have used their mobile phone to share intimate content[2]). So in this scenario we could potentially have a vulnerable minor who is feeling isolated and alone as a result of having sent an image of him or herself which has then been distributed further by the recipient, who has nowhere to turn because their expectation is that they will, at the very least, be told off for having done it, rather than helped. And certainly recent legal discussions on this issue would show that this belief by young people is not without foundation (Stone, 2011).

However, the law can be applied in a sensible manner in some cases. In February 2015, two teenage boys, aged 14 and 15 at the time of the offences, were charged in relation to the possession and distribution of indecent photographs of children after one boy had sold the other photographs sent to him by his ex-girlfriend, who was under 16 at the time (Agate and Phippen, 2015). A successful prosecution resulted in both offenders being given referral orders. This appeared to be a reasonable and pragmatic application of the law, following the ACPO advice. However, public reaction to the case presented worrying social attitudes towards the victim. One of the comments left in response to reporting of the case typifies the attitude still prevalent in many cases in relation to the victims:

> She sent the pictures in the first place, why hasn't she been charged with distributing images? He wouldn't have had any to sell if she hadn't sent them … She started it all the minute she pressed 'send' on that selfie.
>
> (A female poster on a Facebook page
> belonging to a local newspaper)

Around the same time another case showed similar attitudes: John Dale,[3] a drunken student, was filmed by his friend Sam Hobley slapping a sleeping girl's face with his genitals, with the recording subsequently being shared. This also resulted in a proportionate outcome. Hobley's colleagues, who saw the recording, recognized it for what it was – sexual assault – with the offender receiving a prison term of nine months. The friend who recorded the video (and also admitted a related charge of sexual assault) received a sentence of nine months, suspended for two years. However, again public opinion of the case was mixed and in some cases seemed to view the prosecution as overzealous, and the conduct only harmless 'banter'. Again, from a personal perspective when speaking about this case with students in lectures at various universities, and also talking about it with older children in schools, the usual reaction to the description of the act is laughter, before it is pointed out this is actually sexual assault and the offender is now in prison.

This is an attitude that manifests itself at many levels in our society. It seems to demonstrate a view that prohibition is the best approach and victims are perhaps in some way responsible for their own abuse. In a recent ruling on a case where a 19-year-old had coerced a 15-year-old into disclosing increasingly explicit images, backed with threats of public exposure if she did not do as she was asked, the judge ruling in the case, while finding the defendant guilty, also stated: 'We have to protect girls against themselves and teenagers have to realize that conduct of this nature has consequences' (*Peterborough Telegraph*, 2016).

In our work in schools we have heard on many occasions that someone who distributed to further third parties was not being malicious and was perhaps only doing it 'for a laugh'. Even early work in this area, such as Phippen (2009), highlighted that while further distribution was not unusual, most young people surveyed did not think this was done for malicious reasons. Related back to the above quotation from the judge, it is worrying when we observe young people seeing nothing wrong with this, or, as has been our experience a number of times, the belief that the blame for redistribution lies with the victim, who 'shouldn't have sent it out in the first place if they didn't want it to go further'.

Safeguarding via legislation

More recently developed legislation has arisen to try and close the gaps between prosecution of offender and protection of victim. The Criminal Justice and Courts Act 2015 (UK Government, 2015a) was developed, in part, to address the growing issue of 'revenge pornography' which was defined by the Ministry of Justice as 'the sharing of private, sexual materials, either photos or videos, of another person without their consent and with the purpose of causing embarrassment or distress', and applies to material made available both online and offline. Clearly there are parallels here with teen sexting incidents.

During the months of debate and calls for legislative change to tackle the growing problem, it was announced on 12 October 2014 that the Criminal Justice and Courts Bill would create a specific offence of revenge pornography, with the then Justice Secretary Chris Grayling stating an intention to inform 'those who fall victim to this type of disgusting behaviour to know that we are on their side and will do everything we can to bring offenders to justice'.

Specifically within the Act, sections 33 to 35 address the revenge pornography issue. Section 33 of the new Act provides as follows:

Disclosing private sexual photographs and films with intent to cause distress

(1) It is an offence for a person to disclose a private sexual photograph or film if the disclosure is made –

    (a) without the consent of an individual who appears in the photograph or film, and

    (b) with the intention of causing that individual distress.

The key elements of this offence are lack of consent and intention to cause distress. Section 33(8) stipulates that intent will not be found simply because disclosure 'was a natural and probable consequence of the disclosure', i.e. the sending of the image did not result in implied consent for further distribution.

Probably the most significant change brought in by the Act was the increased sentencing power it makes available to the courts for these types of activity, increased from six months to two years, demonstrating how serious the offence is and the impact it can have on the victims. Of further significance is the width of the content protected. A film or photograph is 'private' if it 'shows something that is not of a kind ordinarily seen in public' and 'sexual' not only if it shows explicit content, but if it shows something that a 'reasonable person' would consider to be sexual.[4]

At a similar time, the Serious Crime Bill (UK Government, 2015b) delivered legislation intended to protect young people further from being victims of such activity, inserting a new section into the Sexual Offences Act 2003, which created a new offence of 'sexual communication with a child'. The Bill stated that the offence will be committed where a person above the age of 18 intentionally communicates a sexual communication with an individual they do not reasonably believe to be over 16, for the purposes of sexual gratification; or alternatively, where the communication is intended to elicit a sexual communication from the recipient. A communication is defined as sexual if any part of it relates to sexual activity or where a reasonable person would, in all the circumstances, consider it to be sexual. Again, sentencing guidance highlights the severity of the offence, stating it is punishable by up to two years in prison.

When examining protection mechanisms within the legislative process, playing 'catch up' with technology is never going to result in well thought out, effectively debated statute. Instead we end up with ill-considered and impulsive ad hoc reactions which, while well intentioned, do not explore the greyer areas of social practice. For example, the Serious Crime Bill 2015 made it illegal for an adult to request sexually explicit materials from a minor via technology, which is seemingly on the face of it very sensible. However this fails to acknowledge, for example, a 17-year-old and 15-year-old couple using technology to engage in the more explicit aspects of their relationship at the point at which the older participant turns 18. Could the law be disproportionately applied, to result in the 18-year-old being prosecuted in such a case?

In the case of the Criminal Justice and Courts Act, while one may suggest that this legislation could be applied to the protection of child victims in sexting incidents, the law does not replace the Protection of Child Act 1978, so we do, in essence, have a tension between two pieces of legislation. In the light of this, how can a victim be protected under one piece of legislation if they are viewed as an offender in another?

If we take the perspective of some legislators and law enforcement professionals, as represented in the media, it is interesting to see the difference between protection of the adult and child victim. On the one hand we have calls for minors who engage in the self-generation and distribution of indecent images to be prosecuted. Yet, on the other hand, with the introduction of the new revenge porn laws, we have greater protection than ever for adults who engage in exactly the same practices and get caught out in the same way. This seems like a gross disparity and one that demonstrates how difficult it is to legislate in this area. Even if we could deliver education programmes where young people engaged with the legislative position of the behaviours with which they are engaging – and given the perceived failures prohibitive approaches have had towards issues such as smoking, drinking alcohol, or taking illegal narcotics (Plant and Plant, 1999), we might suggest that such engagement is not likely to be particularly forthcoming – we do not have a clear view with which to reassure the victims that by disclosing abuse there would be legal protection for them. Therefore, it is unsurprising that young people have little confidence with adults successfully resolving issues that arise from sexting.

Filling the safeguarding void

Theoretically we could conclude that a prohibitive, legislative approach to education is best. This would be one where the complexities of the social context need no exploration because victims are simply breaking the law and should stop. However we know this approach to be ineffective at safeguarding children from the risks associated with sexting. We must therefore conclude that to address the harm that can arise from sexting, education needs to go much further than simple prohibition.

Young people need to be aware that while sexting is, in their eyes, normal, it does not mean they are expected to tolerate the resultant abuse that can arise. Victims are rarely to blame for the redistribution of an image. However, we must also be mindful that the behaviour on the part of the supposed offender is often ill conceived and lacking in malice. While it might seem unusual for someone who grew up before the advent of social media to see sending an indecent, unsolicited image as a prelude to genuine friendship, affection, and romance, the dearth of pastoral education in this area means it is not an entirely unreasonable expectation for young people in the twenty-first century, however unwise it might appear to their elders.

Although there is provision in the UK's National Curriculum for such subjects to be discussed and for guidance to be given, Sex and Relationship Education (SRE) and Personal, Social, Health and Economic Education (PSHE) are often seen as inferior to the more academic subjects in most UK schools, with less time given to them and fewer resources. We highlighted in the previous chapter the lack of awareness by staff and governors around these issues, particularly related to what digital technology does to social relationships. We have some sympathy for schools which do not engage readily with these topics, given the lack of statutory requirements and resources. With constant pressure on schools to improve academic attainment, why would senior managers or governors decide to allocate time in the curriculum to something complex, requiring constant updating, and non-compulsory?

However, with increasing calls for effective social, personal, sex, and relationship education, in April 2014, the Education Select Committee announced an inquiry into Personal, Social, Health and Economic Education (PSHE) and Sex and Relationship Education (SRE) in schools, with the following points to address (Education Select Committee, 2015):

- whether PSHE ought to be statutory, either as part of the National Curriculum or through some other means of entitlement
- whether the current accountability system is sufficient to ensure that schools focus on PSHE
- the overall provision of Sex and Relationships Education in schools and the quality of its teaching, including in primary schools and academies

- whether recent government steps to supplement the guidance on teaching about sex and relationships, including consent, abuse between teenagers, and cyber-bullying, are adequate
- how the effectiveness of SRE should be measured

The inquiry took place in the wake of the House of Lords' rejection of compulsory SRE earlier in that year, where an amendment to the Children and Families Bill that would have made Sex and Relationships Education (SRE) mandatory in state-funded schools was rejected (*Pink News*, 2015). It is interesting to note that, in the inquiry report, cyberbullying and sexting were both raised and discussed as aspects of relevant, up-to-date, personal and social development that needed to be explored within these curricula (Education Select Committee, 2015). At the conclusion of the inquiry report it was stated:

> There is a lack of clarity on the status of the subject. This must change, and we accept the argument that statutory status is needed for PSHE, with sex and relationships education as a core part of it. We recommend that the DfE develop a workplan for introducing age-appropriate PSHE and SRE as statutory subjects in primary and secondary schools, setting out its strategy for improving the supply of teachers able to deliver this subject and a timetable for achieving this. The statutory requirement should have minimal prescription content to ensure that schools have flexibility to respond to local needs and priorities. SRE should be renamed relationships and sex education to emphasize a focus on relationships.
>
> Parental engagement is key to maximising the benefits of SRE. The Government should require schools to consult parents about the provision of SRE, and ask Ofsted to inspect the way in which schools do this. The existing right of a parent to withdraw their child from elements of SRE must be retained.
>
> (*ibid.*: 4)

The government response to the inquiry report took some time, however, the Secretary of State of Education did write back to the inquiry chair, Neil Carmichael MP, in January 2016. An excerpt from that letter (Morgan, 2016) is reproduced below:

> The vast majority of schools already make provision for PSHE and while the Government agrees that making PSHE statutory

would give it equal status with other subjects, the Government is concerned that this would do little to tackle the most pressing problems with the subject, which are to do with the variable quality of its provision, as evidenced by Ofsted's finding that 40 per cent of PSHE teaching is less than good. As such, while we will continue to keep the status of PSHE in the curriculum under review, our immediate focus will be on improving the quality of PSHE teaching in our schools.

I want PSHE to be at the heart of a whole-school ethos that is about developing the character of young people. I want it to be tailored to the individual needs of the school and for programmes to be based on the best available evidence of what works. I want senior leaders to ensure that it has the time in the curriculum and the status that it deserves within school and I want it to be taught by well-trained and well-supported staff.

(ibid.)

What the response shows is that the UK Government, at present, has little enthusiasm for the introduction of compulsory PSHE and SRE in schools, let alone any commitment to more detail about what that provision should be. In essence, the response suggests that it is down to individual schools to decide how to deliver SRE and PSHE in their school, with no statutory requirement to do so or national guidance on what to deliver.

However, in contrast to this, around the same time as the response on SRE/PSHE in schools, the Department for Education did launch a consultation on safeguarding in schools, laying out draft guidance on what they expected schools to deliver in this area (Department for Education, 2015). At the time of writing this consultation is still ongoing, and while much of this consultation lies outside of the scope of this discussion, there are some interesting points that highlight both some positive and concerning attitudes towards what online safety should be in schools:

75. As schools and colleges increasingly work online it is essential that children are safeguarded from potentially harmful and inappropriate online material. As such governing bodies and proprietors should ensure appropriate filters and appropriate monitoring systems are in place. Children should not be able to access harmful or inappropriate material from the school or colleges IT system. Governing bodies and proprietors should be confident that systems are in place that will identify

> children accessing or trying to access harmful and inappropriate
> content online.
>
> *(ibid.*: 22)

From the positive perspective, it is encouraging to note that the guidance does acknowledge the fact that safeguarding extends to the digital world. However, it would seem from this paragraph that the focus of this safeguarding is protection from harmful content, rather than protection from abuse that might arise from behaviours such as sexting. It also places the responsibility for this protection squarely with the governing body of the school. As we have highlighted in the previous chapter, we have little confidence that governing bodies are appropriately knowledgeable to understand the nature of these issues, let alone provide scrutiny over a school's senior leadership team to ensure effective practice is in place.

However, perhaps of more concern is that the proposed solution to this safeguarding issue lies in technological intervention – through filtering, to prevent access to such content, and monitoring, to ensure young people do not try to access such material. We will return to this point in the following chapter, where we explore in more detail the over-reliance on technology to ensure safeguarding. However, concern is that, again, a technical system is viewed as something to provide a solution to a problem with a social context.

The document suggests that monitoring will allow concerns to be quickly identified and addressed. In returning to the expectation around education on safeguarding topics, the document expands on this expectation:

> 77. Governing bodies and proprietors should ensure children are
> taught about safeguarding, including online, through teaching
> and learning opportunities, as part of providing a broad and
> balanced curriculum. This may include covering relevant issues
> through personal, social, health and economic education (PSHE),
> and/or – for maintained schools and colleges – through sex and
> relationship education (SRE).
>
> *(ibid.*: 22)

It is encouraging to see that safeguarding education, including online issues, is expected to be delivered in schools. However, we are missing important guidance on the content as well as the practicalities of delivery. In the light of this, it seems the level and quality of education around this topic will remain patchy at best.

What happens when you tackle a safeguarding issue from a position of ignorance?

We began this chapter from the viewpoint that schools need to tackle safeguarding issues that arise from the hyper-connected society, yet may lack the knowledge and support mechanisms to achieve it. Through our discussion we have highlighted that schools are one of many stakeholders within the safeguarding equation. They might be at the front line of safeguarding incidents, as a consequence of sexting, and they might take guidance and support from others, such as legislators and policymakers. Yet a major problem remains. Legislation that will protect victims, punish offenders, and provide effective deterrent, while being mindful of what might arise in the future, is extremely difficult to achieve in the digital world. While it is challenging to predict which technologies will embed into society in the future, and how they will be used in the social context, it is even more problematic to apply comprehensive and complete legislation to protect those most vulnerable from harm. Equally, as we have seen with many other prohibitive ideologies, a position that uses legislation as the foundation of a preventative strategy is rarely effective.

Sexting is a complex issue. It is not simply the case that a child will reach a certain age then decide the best way to obtain a boyfriend or girlfriend is to take an explicit image of themselves and send it to potential partners. The practice of sexting lies in the need to be popular, to have a boyfriend/girlfriend, to be told you look attractive, to show you are 'grown up', and so on. It is unlikely, even when a young person has received an assembly or some classroom time where their teacher or tutor has reminded them that taking and sending such an image is actually breaking the law, that in the split second when the young person decides to press the send button on their mobile device, they will refrain from doing so by being reminded that they might become criminalized as a result. Equally, as a result of said assembly or class, if a young person does press send, and is subsequently abused as a result of the image being redistributed, it is extremely unlikely they will disclose this abuse if they have been told that what they were doing was illegal. Coupled with the lack of education around these matters, and young people's awareness that, in general, their teachers and tutors lack knowledge of these issues, young people turn to peers to resolve harm and mitigate risk. Obviously this is not an ideal situation if we want to develop a consistent, supportive knowledge base for our young people around digital safeguarding issues. We owe young people much more than this. We are failing in the rights of children to receive effective education (UN General Assembly, 1989: Article 29) in that we are failing to engage with the complexity of an area such as sexting, due to a lack of understanding of the topic at the policy and legislative level. As a result of this lack of understanding, we have shown that stakeholders will fall back on these prohibitive approaches, which, as suggested in the Department for Education draft safeguarding guidance (Department for Education, 2015), will generally rely upon technology to ensure protection from harm. A failure to appreciate the complex and social nature of digital harm and abuse means we risk imposing greater levels of technical surveillance and control on our young people. This would all be done in the vain hope that by doing such we will protect them. This idea of a potential safeguarding dystopia is explored in more depth in the next chapter, which also explores the growing reliance on content control, monitoring, and tracking as ways of ensuring our children and young people are safe. In such ways are contemporary childhoods slowly and painstakingly being eroded.

Notes

[1] The Crown Prosecution Service has a 'Full Code Test' which is used to make decisions on whether to move to prosecution. The first phase is the 'Evidence Test', judging whether there is sufficient evidence to prosecute; and the second is the 'Public Interest Test', judging whether it is in the public interest to move to prosecute. See www.cps.gov.uk/publications/code_for_crown_prosecutors/codetest.html (accessed 8 July 2016).

[2] McAfee Love, Relationships & Technology survey, 2014 (Siciliano).

[3] R. v. Dale, Nottingham Crown Court, October 2014.

[4] Section 35 of the Act.

Chapter 6
A safeguarding dystopia

Whenever generational changes in children's safeguarding are discussed, 1940s Enid Blyton novels are usually invoked. In her books, relatively young children (in this case between the ages of 10 and 13) happily go off for hikes by themselves, defend themselves from smugglers, and row boats to remote seaside coves and islands, with nothing more than a packet of matches and a bottle of lemonade to sustain them. This is all done whilst periodically knocking on the doors of strange farmhouses to ask for milk and eggs, as the intrepid children unpack their tents and subsist alone in the woods, experiencing a lifestyle that many modern-day children regard with incredulity. While few parents in the 1940s would have approved of facing down smugglers, quite a few of the other activities they engaged in were more common than they might be now, such as going off unsupervised for the whole day in a group, whittling things with penknives, and playing unsupervised around bodies of water. We have discussed contemporary perceptions of this type of physical risk at length in Chapter 2, and subsequent chapters have mapped out the role of different technologies such as biometrics and databases in relation to defining and creating conceptualizations of childhood. The role of this chapter is therefore to draw together these different threads of analysis in examining children's experiences of digital risk in the modern age.

As we have argued, it is clear information and communication technologies, and related excessive data collection, both have the potential to impact negatively on childhood. This raises two important questions. Just because a system can collect data on a child, does this mean it should? A second question is whether society has had sufficient opportunity to reflect upon the value of such data collection, and whether this is proportional to the impact on the child. If it hasn't, the safeguarding imperative then becomes the controlled influence, in order to ensure that something is seen to be done to protect the child, regardless of what the longer term consequences for the child might be. We are imposing increasing amounts of prohibition and surveillance on our children and young people in order to reassure ourselves we are keeping them safe from harm when, in reality, we have no idea whether it will be able to safeguard them properly. We argue that this represents a safeguarding dystopia, in which privacy is being dangerously eroded.

Bruce Schneier, in his classic essay 'The eternal value of privacy' (Schneier, 2006), considers that erosion of privacy across society as a whole results in a population that devolves to become childlike. As he argues:

> For if we are observed in all matters, we are constantly under threat of correction, judgment, criticism, even plagiarism of our own uniqueness. We become children, fettered under watchful eyes, constantly fearful that – either now or in the uncertain future – patterns we leave behind will be brought back to implicate us, by whatever authority has now become focused upon our once-private and innocent acts. We lose our individuality, because everything we do is observable and recordable.
>
> (*ibid.*)

The concern we have with this statement is that it seems to be implying that children are already monitored, judged, and challenged on their behaviours – the default position is already that children should expect to be 'fettered under watchful eyes'. Our research indicates that this is clearly becoming the case, and in this chapter we explore and analyse this phenomenon.

Children, digital behaviours, and safeguarding

In discussions with children and young people themselves about their privacy, as part of the different research projects we have reported upon earlier, we can see a routine acceptance of monitoring, questioning, and interference. When first questioned about privacy, the usual response, in our experience, is one of lack of concern – they have little data that is valuable, and they can view the benefits of some systems that we might consider impact upon their privacy (for example, the biometric systems discussed in Chapter 3). There is a passivity in their attitudes that is worrying, but perhaps unsurprising given the already established levels of data collection imposed upon them, and the lack of education around rights, data, or privacy.[1]

However, when challenged with a scenario where they might feel their privacy is being violated, we tended to see a strongly defensive reaction – almost as if someone had given them permission to raise objections to abuses of privacy for the first time. In general, the scenario that creates the most discussion is a simple one: we say 'if you're not worried about privacy, please can I have a look at your mobile phone?' It would seem from many discussions that the mobile device, with its assemblage of messages, images, videos, and contacts representing a social location of identity, epitomizes privacy for young people, yet they struggle to identify this until there is a direct challenge to it. In discussion with young people, it would seem that they are confident in protecting their mobile devices: they will generally have PIN codes on them, and they are always with them. However, they are extremely uncomfortable with challenges to this privacy, for example by teachers or parents. In some countries this is happening increasingly frequently.

For example, Part 2 of the UK's 2011 Education Act extended the existing 'stop and search' powers of Section 550ZA of the 1996 Education Act, to allow teaching staff in schools to search a pupil or their possessions without consent if they had reason to believe the individual has, or may, commit a criminal offence. The powers are enhanced to the point that a male member of staff would be allowed to search a female pupil, and their possessions, if they believed that a delay in the search in obtaining a female member of staff might result in serious harm to the pupil or others. The law also granted powers for teachers to confiscate items, including electronic devices, and to be able to examine files and even delete data if they had good reason to do so. To some extent this both resembles and is in contrast to the US situation, where pupils are technically able to invoke the Fourth Amendment to the US Constitution in relation to being searched. The Fourth Amendment guarantees 'the right of the people to be secure in their persons, houses, papers, and effects, against unreasonable searches and seizures'. While a 1985 court case, (New Jersey v. T.L.O., 1985) supported this right, it also concluded that there may be certain occasions in school where it may be appropriate to search pupils, as the school is *in loco parentis*, and the term 'reasonable suspicion' is used to provide for such situations, with very precise conditions being applied to its use. The contrast with the UK situation is that the grounds for searching pupils can be considerably less distinct and carefully defined, and it is here where we see pupils becoming most concerned.

This change in legislation has been key to a shift in the relationship between teachers and pupils. It would seem, from our conversations in focus groups with 98 young people between the ages of 12 and 14 across three research projects, that some teachers are certainly acting indiscriminately on their 'stop and search' powers, and are apparently comfortable with taking a mobile phone and asking the child to unlock it so they can search it in order to make sure they are not doing anything 'criminal'.

Empirical data were drawn from the following:

Table 6.1: Research sampling

Date	Project	Age range	No of participants	Professionals present	Location
March 2015	P1 – Young people's attitudes towards digital privacy	12–13	Group 1 – 12 Group 2 – 12 Mixed gender (50/50) in each	1 teacher 1 teacher	Manchester
September 2015	P2 – Discussion of data collection and monitoring tools in schools	12–13	Group 1 – 14 Group 2 – 10 Mixed gender (50/50) in each	1 teacher 1 teacher/1 police officer*	Cornwall
October 2015	P3 – Biometrics in schools (school 1)	13–14	Group 1 – 10 Group 2 – 10 Mixed gender (50/50) in each	1 teacher 1 teacher	Plymouth
October 2015	P3 – Biometrics in schools (school 2)	13–14	Group 1 – 10 Mixed gender (50/50)	1 teacher	Weston-super-Mare
October 2015	P3 – Biometrics in schools (school 3)	12–13	Group 1 – 10 Group 2 – 10 Mixed gender (50/50) in each	1 teacher 1 teacher	Cornwall

*A police officer was present in his role as a schools' liaison officer who wanted to observe

We have on several occasions heard children talk of the embarrassment of having to sit in a classroom while a teacher goes through the contents on their phone. While they might not have anything criminal on the device, they will have private messages and photographs that they are uncomfortable with others viewing, just as an adult would probably feel in a similar situation. As one 13-year-old member of a focus group told us, 'My teacher went through all my pictures in case there was one of him there and there wasn't'. We should also note that there were no occasions described by our sample where further action was taken against the young person as a result of viewing their mobile device. If our findings are typical, and we believe this is likely, it would seem that the legislation does provide excessive powers to the teacher against a backdrop of safeguarding. During the course of our research, we had a conversation with a police officer when he said he was envious of the powers in the Education Act 2011 given to education professionals, as they far exceeded the stop and search powers he had. In the light of our findings, a more careful legal definition would seem to be advisable, as in the US legislation. There also appears to be considerable confusion about the existing powers amongst young people. When we asked focus groups whether it was acceptable for a teacher to look through the contents of a pupil's phone, responses ranged from, 'it's not their business' to 'they would correct my slang for grammar mistakes' and 'teachers know all about this e-safety stuff and wouldn't go through your phone'. Others were more accepting, telling us that, 'it could be fair', 'they should ask you first', 'teachers – once you are in their classroom you are their responsibility', and 'they should have a proper conversation with you'. Good working relationships and pupil consent would seem to be important to young people, therefore, regardless of what the law says.

One of our teenage research subjects in a secondary school in the south west of England reported another case of excessive surveillance by a teacher that was typical of many we have come across when speaking to focus groups. A 14-year-old girl admitted that she had been answering back in class. The teacher said that her behaviour was unsatisfactory and asked her to step out of the room (an established behaviour management technique in the school). However, after being outside for ten minutes the teacher came to see her and took her into a side room, next to the class, but with no visible linkage, where he produced a digital recording device and proceeded to 'interview' her about her behaviour. In the absence of any parental consent to conduct such an interview, particularly with no supporting adult present, we would very much doubt the legality of this practice, even taking into account the relative vagueness of the 2011 Act.

Yet the child felt powerless to challenge the presence of the recording device, no matter how unsettling its presence might feel to her. Here surveillance was not only excessive, but being used for intimidation, rather than any legitimate safeguarding or child protection concern.

The viewing of mobile devices and use of surveillance, we were told, can also extend into the home. While some young people talked to us about their parents respecting their privacy and only looking at their mobile devices either with permission, or not at all, others said they were subject to 'spot checks' so the parent could be 'reassured' that the child was not doing anything wrong. In a number of cases the young people said their parent said they did this because they cared about their well-being. For example, one pupil told us, 'I make sure my parents know my password' (girl, 13). Young people also describe scenarios in the home where parental concern about mobile devices often extended into other systems, where a parent would receive copies of any communication via messaging apps or SMS. Parents could also view browsing histories, and have remote access to the device, effectively rendering any right to privacy null and void. Occasionally parents also physically tracked their children remotely using GPS. When we asked focus groups about whether this was acceptable behaviour on the part of parents, our young research participants varied in their views, ranging from, 'it is my private phone' (girl, 13), to 'it depends how old the child is' (boy, 13), and in one case 'it would be a bit of a lazy parent' (girl, 13). A more outraged member of the focus group insisted to the others, 'human rights, people! It's your right to go where you have agreed within a specific area!' (boy, 13), and another girl of the same age said, in a very world-weary tone that belied her youth, 'what have we come to, that we have to have trackers on little people's phones?'. When we probed further on when this might be age appropriate, some answered up to Year 6 (age 11 in England and Wales) whereas others thought it should be Years 1–4 (age 5 to 9 in England and Wales), so in this case younger children than the age of the pupils in the focus groups concerned, whose ages were on average around 12–14. Sometimes parents carried out assiduous amounts of surveillance. 'My mum is always checking my phone, especially at night', a 12-year-old boy told us. At other times, parental surveillance didn't always work as planned. 'Mum took my phone for two days to check my texts but none came through', reported one 12-year-old girl, and one 13-year-old boy told us, 'it drained my phone's battery'. Many pupils reported deleting anything to do with medical and body searches (usually involving them trying to find out about matters to do with puberty and sex) from their browsing history. Others were anxious about intrusive and unsolicited advertisements on their phones giving the wrong impression to their parents about what they had been doing with their phones. It was clear to us that families are continually seeking a balance between trying to take advantage of the freedoms that a mobile phone offers, for example the ability to communicate spontaneously and also for parents to know if their children need help, with significant privacy and safeguarding concerns. Parental phones, on the other hand, seemed to be off limits. 'I don't know if it's right to look at my mum's messages', reported one 13-year-old boy.

While we might consider some of these examples to represent excessive surveillance of the child, there is certainly support for it beyond the family situation. Claire Perry, the Conservative MP for Devizes, and at the time of writing the UK Transport Minister, was previously the Prime Minister's Special Adviser on Preventing the Sexualization and Commercialization of Childhood. In a media interview (BBC, 2013) she said that she believed parents should be able to spot check a child's mobile device at any time. She even went as far as saying that the idea that children have a right to keep their personal messages private was 'bizarre'. While Ms Perry might find a child's right to privacy bizarre, we have had children reflecting on the extent of surveillance by parents – one suggesting that given the potential for having the whole school day recorded on a mobile video device, perhaps that would be the logical next step. Would parents spend their entire day viewing the experiences of the child at school, in order to reassure them they weren't swearing, being bullied, or engaging in unsavoury practices? The independent school Queen Ethelburga's College in Yorkshire was subject to criticism from the Independent Schools Inspectorate report recently, having installed over 500 CCTV cameras in order to make every aspect of education visible to those who might wish to see it (Independent Schools Inspectorate, 2015). Might digital parenting take up so much time that there would be little left for anything else, and would the reassurance given by this make it worthwhile?

Yet while we reflected on this practice, those who were subjected to it were already developing their own strategies for maintaining their privacy while assuaging their parents' concerns. Images were not stored on phones, but were immediately uploaded to cloud-based storage, password-protected away from parental eyes. Messages that may be considered inappropriate (to quote one young man: 'why do I hear "inappropriate" so much!?') are removed from the device before going home, or applications are used that aren't placed under the umbrella of the monitoring systems. This is not because anything they were doing was illegal, but simply because young people would rather their parents did not see everything they shared with friends, in the same way their parents wouldn't get to hear every conversation they had in school, or on the school bus at the end of the day. While they could appreciate that this imposition of monitoring was perhaps conducted due to concern, they also felt that such measures were disproportionate and unacceptable, as we have reported. And due to their technical knowledge, and the support of peers, they were working out ways to 'cheat' the systems. As soon as one member of a year group had developed a strategy for bypassing safeguarding systems, the knowledge soon disseminated to peers. In terms of computer science knowledge, we saw situated cognition in action in a collective sense. The skills young people needed to ensure their own privacy were skills developed as they were required. In one sense this is reassuring, in that pupils clearly feel able to carve out private spaces in their digital worlds. On the other hand, such behaviour presents one of the key challenges to an over-reliance on technology to solve what we must view as social problems. Technological solutions can be good at dealing with clearly defined situations (e.g. verifying the existence of credit cards), but not necessarily very effective at dealing with complexity or unpredictability. This can result in not just a digital divide, but also a privacy divide, for some groups within society (House of Commons Home Affairs Committee, 2008).

Block it, monitor it, track it, safeguard it

Content filtering is a well-established tool within the school setting that enables the prevention of access to illegal content (for example, child abuse images) and the control of access to material that might be considered inappropriate for children (for example, pornography, gambling websites, or 'hate' sites). The premise is a simple one: certain types of content could be considered harmful, therefore if we prevent access to such, the harm can be avoided. Filters are, in general, a blunt tool, blocking at either a URL (web address) level (for example, blocking a site such as www.pornhub. com), or searching for blacklisted keywords in the content of the site and making a heuristic-based decision to block based upon occurrence and some limited understanding of the context of those words. So, for example, a word such as 'pornography' would be blocked, whether the content of a pornographic website or an academic essay on the subject was concerned. While we might argue that even an essay on pornography is not something for a child to see, filtering becomes more problematic with more ambiguous words, for example such as 'cock' or 'gay': both have potentially sexual contexts but, equally, they might refer to some other form of content, such as ornithology or happiness. Therefore, filtering software is often criticized for 'over-blocking' – preventing access to perfectly acceptable content based on the judgements of the filter that it contains 'harmful' keywords. This can, obviously, create frustrating browsing experiences for children in their schools, and we have heard many stories about searching for content that was blocked, and that schools are particularly 'risk averse' with blocking levels. One might suggest that this is an example of education professionals needing to manage risk not just in relation to young people, but also to themselves. Internet influences are not alone in their ability to have an adverse effect on children's development (Pardun *et al.*, 2005), but the scope for public censure in the media regarding internet use means it is unsurprising that schools will err on the side of caution. This frequently appeals to teachers, as there is the added potential for pedagogic impact in the classroom, by removing obvious distractions or titillations from the learning environment.

In more recent times, there has been growing concern about access at home and therefore safeguarding thinking has suggested that filtering there might also be necessary. Even as far back as the Byron Review (Byron, 2008) there was much discussion on the advantages and disadvantages of filtering in the home, acknowledging the problems of over-blocking and also issues such as configuration and management. The report did seem to come out on the side of filtering in the home, if managed effectively, calling for industry to ensure such content blocking was available to parents. This is, perhaps, unsurprising, given the focus of the review was harmful and inappropriate content in video games and online. However, during the course of the Byron Review, the scope seemed to expand beyond content-based issues to start referring more broadly to 'online safety' or 'e-safety'. It was therefore no surprise to see filtering becoming the default position for 'child online safety' post-Byron, with both the subsequent UK Coalition Government and today's incumbent administration presenting an ideological position that filtering is the primary issue in protecting children online.

This view has led to a prohibitive policy that has placed the requirement to 'protect' solely in the hands of service providers who should place filtering technologies in the home. This has emerged regardless of concerns raised in the Byron Review that stated that parents needed to engage with dialogue on being safe online rather than becoming complacent because the filter was providing the safety needed in the home. Indeed, it posed the hypothesis that an over-reliance on filters may present a legal challenge against Article 10 of the European Convention on Human Rights (the right to freedom of expression). It also raised concerns about the subjectivity of what could be considered inappropriate.

Over the last few years, a number of parliamentary initiatives, such as Claire Perry's 'Independent parliamentary inquiry into online child protection' (Perry, 2012), David Cameron's speech 'The internet and pornography: The prime minister calls for action' (Cameron, 2013), and Baroness Howe's proposed Private Member's Online Safety Bill[2] (UK Government, 2016) all have, at the core, an expectation that service providers should put tools in place to ensure harmful content cannot be delivered into the home and viewed by children. During this time there has been growing concern over the effectiveness of filtering technologies, with the Open Rights Group launching the Blocked project (Open Rights Group, 2016), which test the top 100,000 websites as defined by the Alexa website ranking project (Alexa, 2016). While results varied depending on the nature of the filtering tool used, they demonstrated that both innocent and useful web content was regularly blocked by these tools. The project also raised personal stories of over-blocking, with a particularly amusing quote from Paul Staines, the editor of the political blog 'Guido Fawkes':

> We would really appreciate it if TalkTalk would remove us from their block list. The only people who block us are them, and the Chinese government.
>
> (cited in Jackson, 2014)

While filtering might be considered annoying or inconvenient for the end user, there is a more damaging impact of over-blocking. Given the dearth of effective sex and relationships education in schools (discussed in Chapter 5) for some young people the internet presents the only opportunity for them to access useful information around sexuality, sexual health, gender identity, and similar issues. All of this sort of content will be blocked by the majority of filtering tools since, given the types of language used in these sites, the keyword matching algorithms of the filters will decide the sites clearly serve up inappropriate content and block them. In this way young people are being prevented from accessing useful, and in some cases much needed, information to help answer the questions they have while growing up. Moreover, when considering the case of young people's rights, we might query the impact of such measures on Article 17 of the United Nations 'Convention on the rights of the child', 'Access to information and mass media' (UN General Assembly, 1990; UNICEF, 2016).

We can also see a challenge from the perspective of 'net neutrality' (Ofcom, 2011), which represents the idea that the internet should not be hampered by discrimination by either service providers or government, and where all data should be treated equally. While much of the net neutrality arguments have focused upon issues such as preferential charging or throttling of services, based upon the type of data being transmitted (for example, reducing capacity on the network when data communicated over peer-to-peer systems is detected), the central premise, that data should not be discriminated against by the service provider before reaching the end user, presents some concerns for filtering. There is even debate over whom the end user might actually be from the perspective of net neutrality. However, if we are to consider the end user to be the individual who has requested the data and wishes to make use of it, rather than the opposing view that the end user is actually the network end point in a domestic setting or the bill payer for the service, filtering does indeed discriminate. While the issues of net neutrality continue to be resolved via legislation, a recent case highlighted a legal perspective against Article 15(1) of the E-Commerce Directive:

> Member States shall not impose a general obligation on providers, when providing the services covered by Articles 12, 13 and 14, to monitor the information which they transmit or store, nor a general obligation actively to seek facts or circumstances indicating illegal activity.
>
> (European Union, 2011)

In a ruling on 24 November 2011 the European Court of Justice ruled in the Scarlet Extended (Belgacom Group) v. Sabam case (*ibid.*) that requiring Internet Service Providers (ISPs) to use systems 'for filtering and blocking electronic communications is inconsistent with EU law'. This case hinged on an injunction on a Belgian ISP attempting to force them to filter content to protect the copyright of the creators and ensure illegal downloads cannot take place. However, the ruling stated that ISPs 'can't be made to install monitoring systems to prevent illegal downloads of copyrighted material'.

The ruling also stated that such monitoring would also 'infringe the fundamental rights of the ISP's customers, namely their freedom to receive or impart information and their right to protection of their personal data and be against the European Convention on Human Rights' (European Union, 2003). It also stated that data must be able to travel 'without discrimination, restriction or interference'.

This ruling seemed very much at odds with the UK Government's perspective on online safeguarding – that service providers are responsible for ensuring homes can filter (and therefore discriminate) amongst data depending upon their nature. However, such is the ideological obsession of the UK Government in terms of ensuring filtering does 'protect children' that this issue was raised in the House of Commons, on 28 October 2015 at

Prime Minister's Questions. When questioned on the EU ruling, the Prime Minister stated:

> Like my hon. Friend, I think that it is vital that we enable parents to have that protection for their children from this material on the internet. Probably like her, I spluttered over my cornflakes when I read the *Daily Mail* this morning, because we have worked so hard to put in place those filters. I can reassure her on this matter, because we secured an opt-out yesterday so that we can keep our family-friendly filters to protect children. I can tell the House that we will legislate to put our agreement with Internet companies on this issue into the law of the land so that our children will be protected.
>
> (Hansard, 2015)

This placed the UK at odds with the European Court ruling and, one might infer, at odds with net neutrality as a concept, against a backdrop of claiming that compromising the pro-filtering position would result in 'our children' not being protected from the dangers of the internet.

However, within this filtering debate, we must return to the central position – that filtering is necessary to ensure children cannot be harmed by inappropriate content. While filtering is a useful tool to prevent accidental access by a younger child, our discussions with young people would suggest that for the determined teenager, who wishes to access 'inappropriate' content, it will fail in its aim. For one, young people know ways around filters – they have a long track record of doing so in school systems, so why would it be any different for filtering at home? But also, perhaps more crucially, the world wide web is but one route to pornography for those wishing to seek it out. Filters will only ever work for pornography (and other content) accessed via a browser. It cannot prevent imagery embedded within other sites (for example, if pornographic images are posted on a social media page), unless the site is blocked in its entirety (which would be doomed to fail in a home filtering scenario). It will also not prevent content that is shared in peer-to-peer systems, via mobile devices, over personal networks (for example, via Bluetooth), and so on. Filtering is supposed to solve the problem of online safety, but it fails to do this even in the most limited sense.

Nevertheless, the reliance on technology to achieve safeguarding goals continues unabated. More recently, arguably driven by the anti-radicalization agenda (UK Government, 2011) another class of system is gaining greater interest from the policymakers – network and internet monitoring tools. These tools play an active role in the interception and analysis of traffic across a network, whether this is when a user tries to access a certain site or, increasingly, flagging warnings to system administrators when certain key phrases are communicated in, for example, messages between two end users. Monitoring systems claim to address a number of safeguarding concerns that cannot be tackled with filtering – those that fall broadly into issues such as cyberbullying and radicalization. If a monitoring system is set up with a catch list to trap aggressive or offensive words between those communicating it can, arguably, raise alerts about potential abuse that can then be addressed in the wider school setting. Monitoring is also sometimes seen as an alternative to aggressive filtering, a means of avoiding the annoyance of over-blocking. In these cases the site might not be blocked (although some joint monitoring and filtering systems will do this) but an alert is raised for an administrator to take investigative action.

The recent draft statutory guidance on safeguarding by the Department for Education (2015), defines an expectation that schools have monitoring in place and the governing body is responsible for it to be 'appropriate'.

> [Schools] need to have appropriate filters and monitoring systems, so that no child can access harmful content via the school's IT systems and concerns can be spotted quickly.
>
> (Department for Education, 2015)

However, there seems to be little guidance on what 'appropriate' means aside from further guidance to ensure 'unreasonable restrictions' are not placed on what can be taught:

> 78. Whilst it is essential that governing bodies and proprietors ensure that appropriate filters and monitoring systems are in place; they should be careful that 'over blocking' does not lead to unreasonable restrictions as to what children can be taught with regards to online teaching and safeguarding.
>
> (*ibid.*)

This does seem somewhat contradictory – on the one hand they are saying governing bodies are responsible for ensuring safeguarding systems are in place in order to protect young people from trying to access inappropriate material or capture offensive communications, but on the other also requiring that systems should not be so restrictive that young people are hampered from accessing legitimate, educational, websites. As can be seen from the discussion around filtering and the Blocked project above, if the combined technical capabilities of the four major ISPs are failing to achieve the balance between protection and over-blocking, it seems like a high expectation to place upon governors. We have already discussed, through the exploration of the 360 Degree Safe data, that governing bodies rarely receive training in these topics and such issues can have complex implications for education, data protection, and privacy.

What is also lacking from the (albeit draft) guidance is any advice on how to deal with alerts when they are raised, or how to resolve issues that may be ambiguous in nature. For example, if school systems detect a child looking at self-harm or sexual health sites, to whom is this disclosed? Are parents informed? And how is the young person's privacy considered – perhaps they are accessing the sites at school because they do not wish for their parents to see that they are looking at sites of this nature? The call to have systems in place with no guidance on how they might be used proportionately raises further concerns around the erosion of children's rights. Again, someone taking a 'safeguarding dystopia' position would argue that, in the face of protection against radicalization, cyberbullying, and inappropriate content, we may have to reduce or preclude some fundamental rights – the balance of rights against protection/safety is a delicate one, and arises in a lot of debates around data surveillance (for example, the Home Office's Investigatory Powers Bill 2015–16, currently being debated at the time of writing). However, without effective guidance around how monitoring may be handled, compounded with legislative expectation for schools to 'do something' with monitoring, and the expectation through the Prevent duty that schools should immediately report any concerns around radicalization, we would expect to see further stories such as a recent case of a school reporting a child to the police when their monitoring systems caught him accessing the website of the UK Independence Party (BBC, 2016).

What is missing from this guidance is advice about the requirement for consent for the collection, use, and storage of a child's data and how incident response is managed. Clearly their browsing habits and potential communications under school systems would need to be covered by this. The schools would also have a responsibility to ensure that the data was protected and that appropriate security was in place for these systems. Again, given our analysis of the 360 Degree Safe database, we are less than confident that all schools have the capabilities to ensure this level of data protection is in place.

Track your child, sleep soundly at night

Outside schools, we are seeing an increasing number of companies offering parents reassurance about the safety of their children with a number of technological interventions, such as monitoring of mobile devices, remote control of computers, and location tracking systems. With location tracking, the technology within mobile devices is exploited so its location can be determined with appropriate software. Of course, these systems are marketed to reassure parents' concerns, assuming that, if you can see where your child is the whole time, there is no need to worry.

The software applications can fall into a number of different categories:

- **Filtering and access control**: to restrict access to web content with filtering; to control when or for how long they can go online
- **Monitoring and interception**: to keep track of SMS messaging and content, emails, and other forms of communication with systems that will either log them or deliver a copy to the parents' device; to set alerts when profanity or words on a 'watch list' are used
- **Remote control of devices**: to access the device or disable it (for example, if a child is not returning calls, the parent can disable the phone as punishment)
- **Location tracking**: to keep track of where a mobile device is using GPS technology
- **Location control**: to make parts of a town (for example, near a river or railway) off limits and receive alerts if a mobile device goes near those areas.

By way of illustration, one product's marketing material promotes all manner of surveillance techniques:

- Monitor with whom my child chats on Facebook
- Block harmful content from search results
- Limit the time kids spend online or on their devices
- Restrict games or applications in their devices
- Track my child's mobile device
- Get Emergency Alerts when my child is in trouble
- Block or monitor calls and SMS activity
- Prevent kids from accessing mature or adult sites
- Protect and monitor more than one child at one time
- View and manage their activities from anywhere
- Protect and monitor without my kids knowing

(Qustodio, 2016)

Perhaps in this list of child surveillance and control technologies, the final point is the most sinister: why would a parent wish to monitor their child without them knowing? Surely that presents long-term trust issues that would not easily be resolved once a child discovered the surveillance. The concept of 'covert protection' is highly concerning.

In terms of parental response, danah boyd [sic] has reflected upon this in discussions with parents through her own ethnographic research (boyd, 2014) with one parent telling her:

> I do not believe that teenagers need privacy, not when it comes to the internet. I track everything my kids do online. I search their bedrooms too. I'm the parent, I'm not their friend.
>
> (*ibid.*: 71)

Another parent interviewed for a newspaper article, who used remote tracking and monitoring application (including video surveillance technology in the home) as he worked away from the family home during the week, felt that the technologies brought him reassurance:

> I am away far more than I'd like to be; my wife takes care of our two teenage children but I want to know what's going on and now the technology exists to achieve this. If I ring and ask her what she's up to, I like to know she's telling the truth. I know it's a bit heavy, but as a parent working away from home, I want to feel in control. For me it's about escalation. Teenagers today have the technology to lead hidden lives. I need new gadgets to keep up.
>
> (Odell, 2014)

From our own experiences, there are certainly parents who believe that monitoring their children, either explicitly or covertly was the right thing to do. In one instance a parent told us that while her daughter did not yet have a mobile phone, when she did she would be demanding random spot checks to ensure she was not misbehaving. Again, she used reassurance as a justification of this – if she could see her daughter's phone and reassure herself she was behaving, she could trust her. However, how she might break out of this trust/reassurance/monitoring cycle was unclear.

Perhaps the most extreme example of parental surveillance that we have come across was a parent whose 14-year-old daughter had become concerned about the behaviour of her friend, who had recently started a relationship that the daughter feared was sexual. The parent asked her daughter to access her friend's Facebook account (by fraudulently obtaining her password) so they could read the messages that she had sent to her boyfriend and, once they had discovered some message with sexual connotations, they arranged an 'intervention' for the girl, justified because the parent 'would never have forgiven herself' if the friend had become pregnant.

Keeping children 'safe' online

Technology is now available that could potentially track and collect data on how young people use digital technology, how they interact with peers, what sorts of information they look for, and where they are, throughout their whole day. Will this provide reassurance for parents and ensure that their children are safe from the 'dangers' of the internet? Schools can collect data on young people to fulfil the growing statutory requirements being placed upon them to ensure their safeguarding responsibilities. But will this safeguarding dystopia actually achieve its aims in making sure children and young people cannot come to any harm? We would suggest that chasing social problems with technology will ultimately not create a safe environment for young people, but will instead create an atmosphere of mistrust, tensions between adults and young people, and the development of a generation who have their rights to access information, relevant and up-to-date education, and privacy eroded, while it is argued that it's for their own good.

This raises a number of questions. For example, does surveillance, monitoring, and tracking actually reassure anyone? While it might initially be reassuring to be able to see where a child is, based upon the location tracking on their mobile device, what happens when we realize that this software is providing access to the location of the mobile device, not the young person? What if they have left the device with a friend? What happens if the device loses coverage? Or the software fails? In discussing this issue with young people, they have raised all of these questions – but they have also raised other concerns, for example: 'What about our human rights?'

In the projects reported earlier, we also discussed with young people whether such technology can provide reassurance in a relationship (for example, if a partner asks to track an individual's mobile to reassure them because they are feeling insecure). While some initially would suggest that they could not see much wrong with this, peers would raise all sorts of different issues to challenge this passivity. They make observations such as that if that is the foundation for trust in a relationship, then it is not worth having.

It would seem from our discussions that young people believe that tracking and monitoring technology does not provide reassurance, but creates anxiety and mistrust. By way of simple example, we have written on many occasions about the messaging application WhatsApp, which allows the sender of a message to know whether the message has been sent (one grey tick), has been received (two grey ticks), and has been viewed by the recipient (two blue ticks). Many of them talk about the stress from the 'two blue ticks' if the recipient doesn't reply, or they say they haven't seen a message when the app says they have. The app can also show whether a recipient is online or not, again adding to anxiety if the conversation doesn't keep flowing. There is a greater issue around trust between the adult and the child. Covert surveillance is rarely an effective way to build trust, regardless of the good intentions of the adult. And if there is no trust in the relationship, if a young person does get into some trouble (for example, a sexting incident), it is extremely unlikely that they would disclose the abuse or harm to an adult they didn't trust (as discussed in the previous chapter). And such a scenario would be entirely possible even with a whole raft of monitoring technologies – children could obtain devices their parents weren't aware of, or they could use unmonitored platforms: they will find a way if they want to.

We must also reflect upon the motivations of companies producing these technologies. They are preying on the anxieties of parental insecurity to provide reassurance they will sell for a profit. Of course they will sell the technology with lots of positive messages about reassurance and care. It is unlikely that such a product would be as successfully marketed with a strapline of 'erode your children's rights and gain empty reassurances about their online safety'. Technology is now sufficiently advanced that all manner of surveillance is possible, but just because we can, does that mean we should? Within the school setting, and at home, we are developing a society where we are forgetting about the essentials for building effective relationships, such as trust, knowledge building, and shared experiences. What sort of a society are we moving towards where 'trust' relies on surveillance and data collection? We are failing to reflect upon the impact on young people if they are told every move, every message, and every website access is collected and they are queried on every aspect. In the analogue age the best a parent might have expected from a question such as 'how was school?' was generally a response like 'boring', or 'it was OK'. Without intense digital surveillance, on the whole children still managed to develop into intelligent well-adjusted adults.

If we return to the UN 'Convention on the rights of the child' (UN General Assembly, 1990), we can very clearly see that our safeguarding dystopia presents challenges against:

- Article 17 (access to information; mass media)
- Article 29 (goals of education)
- Article 34 (sexual exploitation)

With more complex data collection, monitoring, and surveillance, we would also suggest the following are challenged:

- Article 12 (respect for the views of the child)
- Article 13 (freedom of expression)
- Article 16 (right to privacy)

And, more widely, we should also consider:

- Article 42 (knowledge of rights)

To be a young person in the twenty-first century means living a cloistered and constrained digital life. This is because it is easier – and cheaper – for us to introduce indiscriminate prohibition rather than tackle the root cause of offensive material and interaction on the internet. Hence we are moving into a world where children's rights are increasingly eroded, with the perennial justification of child safety seen as a catch-all for any measure that any single group deems necessary, whether this is democratic in origin or not. This political, commercial, and domestic obsession with data collection and tracking of individuals is coupled with a dearth of education around the impact of technology on society, digital rights, and relationship and sex education. This means our young people risk failing to develop any proper awareness of their or others' rights. In almost all situations, we have found they have restricted access to information, limited agency, and are more often than not, unable to express themselves freely. That hardly sounds like the foundations for a next generation of responsible well-informed adults.

Notes

[1] While the National Curriculum for England current at the time of writing (www.gov.uk/government/collections/national-curriculum) has some expectation of education around 'online safety', reinforced with the most recent inspectorate framework, which places challenges around this area (Ofsted, 2016), there is little evidence, in our experience, that young people in England get much opportunity to discuss and debate the complexities of privacy and safety/security. It is more likely they are simply told to 'think before you post' in case actions come back to haunt them in the future.

[2] 'A Bill to make provision about the promotion of online safety; to require ISPs and mobile phone operators to provide an internet service that excludes adult content; to require electronic device manufacturers to provide a means of filtering internet content; to make provision for parents to be educated about online safety and for the regulation of harmful material through on-demand programme services' (UK Government, 2016).

Chapter 7

A manifesto

It has never been safer to be a child than in the twenty-first century. Thanks to global increases in GDP over the last 150 years, we have seen the growth of free universal education, the development of extensive pre-natal and paediatric healthcare provision, the introduction of population-based vaccination programmes, increasing tolerance of difference, and extensive recognition of children's rights. This has meant that for many children, in the West at least, childhood can be relatively long in duration, spent mainly engaging in education, with ample leisure time. Yet it is clear from our experience of talking to children, parents, and teachers that it does not feel as though childhood represents a period of freedom from the pressures that are likely to be experienced as adults. Instead, contemporary childhood takes many forms simultaneously, presenting conflicting models at the same time. Children are seen as immature and ignorant in that they cannot make judgements about technology, but also threatening in that they might engage in cyberbullying. They are innocents, seen as unable to make appropriate choices, but they are expected to take responsibility for transmitting sexual content via social media. They are heavy consumers of digital hardware, software, and social media platforms, and actively marketed to, yet they are increasingly criticized for spending their lives experiencing a socially constructed existence through the medium of a computer screen.

Within this confused terrain, we see many aspects of twenty-first-century post-industrial politics reflected. The trend towards globalization has meant that national data protection laws and protocols have become increasingly challenged. Large numbers of international stakeholders are involved in redefining childhood across the public and private sectors, and a number of dominant interests prevail, such as the involvement of multinational corporations in education and domestic life. The concept of human rights has become less abstract and increasingly tightly defined in different contexts, leaving areas that are difficult to define unresolved (such as the right to enjoy aspects of an analogue life in an increasingly digital world). The role of social membership and identity in everyday life has shifted, moving from one where we might have experienced a small number of deep relationships to one where hundreds of relatively shallow ones represent the norm. All this has meant that new social inequalities have proliferated for children, and individual freedoms have been constrained in new ways.

While childhood has always brought with it various forms of ascribed status, and particular sets of expectations, the confusion surrounding the contemporary definition of childhood means that it is all too easy for modern children to fall foul of rapidly shifting, paradoxical, and often unintelligible social expectations. These are rarely properly articulated in a manner that young people can fully understand and engage with. We have established that twenty-first-century children access technology for two main reasons: voluntarily (for social networking and gaming purposes) and involuntarily (for identity and administration purposes). Yet despite the best efforts of schools it can be difficult for children to recognize the boundaries between the two, and there can be undesirable consequences if the categories are confused or blurred, as is often the case in our hyper-connected society. This is because within a consumer society, there is a gradual move away from 'the real' towards increasing levels of simulation of the real, indicated by particular signs and symbols, as argued by Baudrillard (1994). This brings with it significant philosophical and ethical issues, particularly in the cases of sexting and surveillance of children at school. The penalty for misunderstanding these signs and symbols, or failing to appreciate them properly, can be harsh, at best what sociologists might classify as a spoiled identity, where an individual may become the brunt of many punishments, criticism, or jokes at his or her expense, but at worst it can culminate in spurious criminal records or at the very extreme end, as we have seen, young people taking their own lives.

Key to understanding this as a social problem is recognizing the risks associated with technology being imposed upon children, such as the use of biometrics in schools and surveillance software being deployed without their consent or even knowledge. Here technology serves multiple functions as a proxy for efficiency and modernization of school systems, yet the kind of panoptical digital surveillance many children experience today has the potential for considerable harm in the manner described above. This is because in such cases, human relationships have become subservient to machine-based ones. With this in mind, we have discussed the impact of such technology use on the identity and privacy rights of children. The prevalence of such strong levels of technology in many schools, as well as the hyper-connected nature of children's lives outside school that we have described, mean that teachers are ill equipped to monitor and guide children and young people in their attempts to navigate an increasingly complex society, as we have seen in our various research findings. Until schools and other educational settings adapt their pedagogic practices in order to address what is by any standard a fundamental societal shift, the danger is that many children will continue to be blighted by its effects, and consequently certain undesirable behaviours such as violence, disaffection, and certain forms of social inequality will be normalized.

In practical terms, we argue that the lived experience of these technologies suggests that it is time for a revised national (or indeed international) curriculum dealing more effectively with the role of technology within everyday life. This also has implications for the way schools and other organizations should interact with children in terms of technology. We see such a curriculum as going well beyond the current limited diet of online safety and computer coding, instead embracing topics such as:

- privacy, information, and education rights
- management of time and space
- the provision, maintenance, and protection of digital infrastructure
- the role of technology within relationships
- digital criminology
- digital citizenship
- digital consumption
- respect, consent, and empathy with others
- legislative protections
- the role of media as information source and influencer
- well-being and mental health

These are all vitally important topics to address at this point in human history. The technology industry continues to experience exponential growth, thanks to increasing processing power and general affordability issues. Companies are therefore pushing social networking, gaming, and biometric products hard within a comparatively mature market, including to schools, in an attempt to ensure market share and profitability for the future. They are also keen to purchase personal data collected by public bodies such as healthcare providers and educational institutions, in order to feed this business model further. We are moving towards fresh debates on artificial intelligence and robotics, and in years to come, new issues are likely to be raised, ranging from digital biology via implants to power supply and reliability issues, the impact of virtual reality upon the physical world, and potentially even new forms of human reproduction. Penetration of digital issues into the everyday lives of children and their families, along with the associated hyperreality, is likely to continue to grow as a concern. At the same time we have seen stakeholders in children's welfare struggle to keep up with the impact of the digital upon childhood and responding in a reactive and disproportionate way. As we have discussed in this book, there are many in the political world that believe children's rights have to be eroded in order to make them 'safe' when they engage with technology. We would argue that these responses, whose attitudes towards young people's rights are more nineteenth century than modern day, arise from a failure to appreciate the role digital technology plays in young people's lives and a lack of understanding of the active nature of this. In a hyper-connected world, children should be encouraged to demand greater rights to privacy, to information, and to data protection, and not give them up to whichever adult decides they know best. Otherwise we risk the next generation being one that has little understanding of how human rights sit alongside the use of technology. Just because something is technically possible, it does not necessarily mean it should be implemented. If we develop a generation with little awareness of digital moralities, there is a great likelihood that abuses by industry and governments will increase and further erode the rights of the population as a whole.

In response, we need to equip the next generation much more carefully to live within an information age. There is an urgent need to develop an education environment in which children can navigate through the complexity of a connected world. They need to be able to ask questions and ask for help in a supportive, non-judgemental environment. ICT and digital issues should not be subjects that are walled into a specific area of the curriculum – from mathematics to sex and relationship education, there are few aspect of a child's development that do not have some influence from the digital world. To place all of the curriculum attention on technology is as bizarre as placing a topic such as drugs awareness in the chemistry class. This then needs to be supported by policy, practice, and national coordination that acknowledges, rather than shies away from, the challenges that arise from growing up in the twenty-first century. That policy needs to be informed from an evidence base that understands these complex and nuanced issues, rather than being driven by media pressure and gut reaction. This means acknowledging much more fully what it means to be human in a digital world.

References

ACPO (n.d.) *ACPO CPAI Lead's Position on Young People Who Post Self-Taken Indecent Images*. Online. https://ceop.police.uk/Documents/ceopdocs/externaldocs/ACPO_Lead_position_on_Self_Taken_Images.pdf (accessed 8 July 2016).

Agate, J. and Phippen, A. (2015) 'New social media offences under the Criminal Justice and Courts Act and Serious Crime Bill: The cultural context'. *Entertainment Law Review*, 26 (3), 82–7.

Alexa (2016) 'Actionable analytics for the web'. Online. www.alexa.com (accessed 8 July 2016).

Apple, M. (2010) 'The measure of success'. In Monahan, T. and Torres, R. (eds) *Schools under Surveillance*. New Brunswick, NJ: Rutgers University Press.

Ariès, P. (1962) *Centuries of Childhood: A social history of family life*. New York: Knopf.

Ashborne, J. (2000) *Biometrics: Advanced identity verification*. New York: Springer.

Association of British Insurers (2012) 'Time to put the brake on the UK's exorbitant legal bill says the ABI'. Press Release. 23 February. Online. www.abi.org.uk/News/News-releases/2012/02/Time-to-put-the-brake-on-the-UKs-exorbitant-legal-bill-says-the-ABI (accessed 5 July 2016).

A Thin Line (2011) '2011 AP-MTV digital abuse study'. Online. www.athinline.org/pdfs/MTV-AP_2011_Research_Study-Exec_Summary.pdf (accessed 8 July 2016).

Backett-Milburn, K. and Harden, J. (2004) 'How children and their families construct and negotiate risk, safety and danger'. *Childhood*, 11 (4), 429–47.

Barber, M. (1997) *The Learning Game: Arguments for an educational revolution*. London: Indigo.

Barton, A.H. (1969) *Communities in Disaster: A sociological analysis of collective stress situations*. New York: Doubleday.

Baudrillard, J. (1983) *In the Shadow of the Silent Majorities*. Boston: MIT Press.

— (1994) *Simulacra and Simulation*. Ann Arbor: University of Michigan Press.

BBC (2013) 'MP says parents should check their children's messages'. 22 January. Online. www.bbc.co.uk/newsbeat/article/21143662/mp-says-parents-should-check-their-childrens-messages (accessed 8 July 2016).

— (2016) 'Hampshire school calls police after pupil looks at UKIP website'. 28 February. Online. www.bbc.co.uk/news/uk-england-hampshire-35671519 (accessed 8 July 2016).

Beck, U. (1992) *Risk Society: Towards a new modernity*. London: Sage.

— (2007) *World at Risk*. Cambridge: Polity.

Beckford, M. (2012) 'CRB checks top 30 million but create "atmosphere of mistrust"'. *Daily Telegraph*, 23 April.

Big Brother Watch (2014) *Biometrics in Schools: The extent of biometrics in English secondary schools and academies*. London: Big Brother Watch.

Boas, G. (1966) *The Cult of Childhood*. London: Warburg.

Boyce, T., Nellis, M., Corrigan, A.J., Gallagher, H.G., Lee, P., and Sercombe, H. (2010) 'Biometric surveillance in schools: Cause for concern or case for curriculum?'. *Scottish Educational Review*, 42 (1), 3–22.

boyd, d. [sic] (2014) *It's Complicated: The social lives of networked teens*. New Haven, CT: Yale University Press.

Brenner, R.A., Trumble, A.C., Smith, G.S., Kessler, E.P., and Overpeck, M.D. (2001) 'Where children drown, United States, 1995'. *Pediatrics*, July, 108 (1), 85–9.

Brown, M.R. (ed.) (2002) *Picturing Children: Constructions of childhood between Rousseau and Freud*. Aldershot: Ashgate.

Buckingham, D. (2000) *After the Death of Childhood: Growing up in the age of electronic media*. Oxford: Blackwell.

Bunge, M.J. (ed.) (2001) *The Child in Christian Thought*. Grand Rapids, MI: Eerdmans.

Byron, T. (2008) *Safer Children in a Digital World*. London: HMSO.

Calvert, K. (1992) *Children in the House: The material culture of early childhood, 1600–1900*. Boston: Northeastern University Press.

Cameron, D. (2013) 'The internet and pornography: Prime Minister calls for action'. Speech to the National Society for the Prevention of Cruelty to Children. 22 July. Online. www.gov.uk/government/speeches/the-Internet-and-pornography-prime-minister-calls-for-action (accessed 8 July 2016).

Cannella, G. and Kincheloe, J.L. (eds) (2002) *Kidworld: Childhood studies, global perspectives, and education*. New York: Peter Lang.

Clarke, R. (1991) 'Information technology and dataveillance'. In Dunlop, C. and Kling, R. (eds) *Controversies in Computing*. San Diego, CA: Academic Press.

Cleverley, J. and Phillips, D.C. (1986) *Visions of Childhood: Influential models from Locke to Spock*. New York: Teachers College.

Cohen, S. (2002) *Folk Devils and Moral Panic*. Oxford: Routledge.

CPS (n.d.) *Guidelines on Prosecuting Cases Involving Communications Sent via Social Media*. Online. www.cps.gov.uk/legal/a_to_c/communications_sent_via_social_media/ (accessed 8 July 2016).

Cross, G. (1997) *Kids' Stuff: Toys and the changing world of american childhood*. Cambridge, MA: Harvard University Press.

Cunningham, H. (1995) *Children and Childhood in Western Society since 1500*. London: Longman.

Curtis, A., Exley, S., Saisa, A., Tough, S., and Whitty, G. (2008) *The Academies Programme: Progress, problems and possibilities: A report for the Sutton Trust*. London: Institute of Education and Sutton Trust.

Daily Mail (2012) 'Sex texts epidemic: Experts warn sharing explicit photos is corrupting children'. 10 December. Online. www.dailymail.co.uk/news/article-2246154/Sex-texts-epidemic-Experts-warn-sharing-explicit-photos-corrupting-children.html (accessed 8 July 2016).

Daily Telegraph (2003) 'NSPCC's wrong priorities'. 25 February.

Darroch, A. (2011) 'Freedom and biometrics in UK schools'. *Biometric Technology Today*, July/August, 5–8.

Deleuze, G. (1992) 'Postscript on the societies of control'. *OCTOBER*, 59, 3–7.

Department for Education (2015) 'Draft: Keeping children safe in education: Statutory guidance for schools and colleges'. Online. www.gov.uk/government/ uploads/system/uploads/attachment_data/file/487799/Keeping_children_safe_ in_education_draft_statutory_guidance.pdf (accessed 8 July 2016).

Department of Archaeology, Durham University (2012) 'Hand stencils in Upper Palaeolithic cave art'. Online. www.dur.ac.uk/archaeology/research/projects/ all/?mode=project&id=640 (accessed 5 July 2015).

Dombrowsky, W.R. (1989) *Katastrophen und Katastrophenschutz: Eine soziologische analyse*. Wiesbaden: Deutscher Universitatsverlag.

Dombrowsky, W.R. (1998) 'Again and again: Is a disaster what we call a disaster?'. *International Journal of Mass Emergencies and Disasters*, 13, 241–54.

Douglas, M. and Wildavsky, A. (1983) *Risk and Culture: An essay on the selection of technological and environmental dangers*. Berkeley, CA: University of California Press.

Dowty, T. (2008) 'Pixie-dust and privacy: What's happening to children's rights in England?'. *Children & Society*, 22, 393–9.

Doyle, M. (2009) *Children, Consumerism and the Moral Good*. New York: Lexington Books.

Elliott, J. (1996) 'School effectiveness research and its critics: Alternative visions of schooling'. *Cambridge Journal of Education*, 26 (2), 199–223.

Elliott, S.J., Peters, J.L., and Rishel, T.J. (2004) 'An introduction to biometrics technology: Its place in technology education'. *Journal of Industrial Teacher Education*, 41 (4), n.p.

European Union (2003) European Convention on Human Rights Act 2003. Act Number 20.

— (2011) Judgment of the Court (Third Chamber) of 24 November. Case C-70/10. European Court Reports 2011-00000 ECLI identifier: ECLI:EU:C:2011.

Formanek-Brunell, M. (1993) *Made to Play House: Dolls and the commercialization of American girlhood, 1830–1930*. New Haven, CT: Yale University Press.

Furedi, F. (2014) 'NSPCC: Not in the best interests of the child'. *Spiked*, 9 July. Online. www.frankfuredi.com/article/nspcc_not_in_the_best_interests_of_the_ child (accessed 5 July 2016).

Furnham, A. and Gunter, B. (1998) *Children as Consumers: A psychological analysis of the young people's market*. London: Routledge.

Giddens, A. (1991) *Modernity and Self-Identity: Self and society in the late modern age*. Cambridge: Polity.

Goffman, E. (1959) *The Presentation of Self in Everyday Life*. New York: Anchor.

Graham, J.D., Huber, P., and Litan, P. (1991) *The Liability Maze*. Washington: Brookings Institute Press.

Greven, P. (1991) *Spare the Child: The Religious roots of punishment and the psychological impact of physical abuse*. London: Knopf Doubleday.

Hansard (2015) Engagements (Prime Minister's Question Time). Vol. 601. 28 October. Online. http://goo.gl/yO9Vru (accessed 8 July 2016).

Higonnet, A. (1998) *Pictures of Innocence: The history and crisis of ideal childhood*. London: Thames and Hudson.

Hillman, M., Adams, J., and Whitelegg, J. (1988) *One False Move...: A study of children's independent mobility*. London: Policy Studies Institute.

Hope, A. (2007) 'Panopticism, play and the resistance of surveillance: Case studies of the observation of student internet use in UK schools'. *British Journal of Sociology of Education*, 26 (3), 359–73.

Horton, R. (2004) 'UNICEF leadership 2005–2015: A call for strategic change'. *The Lancet*, 364 (9451), 2071–4.

House of Commons Home Affairs Committee (2008) *A Surveillance Society? Fifth Report of Session 2007–08*. Vol. 2: *Oral and written evidence*. Online. www.publications.parliament.uk/pa/cm200708/cmselect/cmhaff/58/58ii.pdf (accessed 22 February 2017).

Huffington Post (2014) 'Sexting could earn teenagers criminal record and a place on Sex Offenders' Register'. Online. www.huffingtonpost.co.uk/2014/07/23/sexting-teenagers-criminal-records_n_5612399.html (accessed 8 July 2016).

Independent Schools Inspectorate (2015) 'Emergency visits report: Queen Ethelburga's College and the Faculty of Queen Ethelburga'. Online. http://media.qe.org/pdf/2015/june-2015.pdf (accessed 8 July 2016).

Information Commissioner's Office (ICO) (2007) *The Guide to Data Protection*. Online. https://ico.org.uk/media/for-organisations/guide-to-data-protection-2-7.pdf (accessed 22 February 2017).

— (2008) 'The use of biometrics in schools'. Statement, August 2008.

— (2015) 'Taking photographs in schools'. Online. https://ico.org.uk/media/for-organisations/documents/1136/taking_photos.pdf (accessed 5 July 2016).

Jackson, M. (2014) 'UK ISP TalkTalk coughs to censorship of political blogger Guido Fawkes'. 2 July. Online. www.ispreview.co.uk/index.php/2014/07/uk-isp-talktalk-coughs-censorship-political-blogger-guido-fawkes.html (accessed 8 July 2016).

James, A., Jenks, C., and Prout, A. (1998) *Theorizing Childhood*. Cambridge: Polity Press.

James, A. and Prout, A. (2004) *Constructing and Reconstructing Childhood: Contemporary issues in the sociological study of childhood*. London: Taylor and Francis.

Kincaid, J.R. (1992) *Child-Loving: The erotic child and Victorian culture*. New York: Routledge.

Kindt, E. (2007) 'Biometric applications and the data protection legislation'. *Datenschutz und Datensicherheit*, 31 (3), 166–70.

Kyriakides, L. and Campbell, R.J. (2004) 'School self-evaluation and school improvement: A critique of values and procedures'. *Studies in Educational Evaluation*, 30 (1), 23–36.

Lacohee, H., Crane, S., and Phippen, A. (2006) *Trustguide: Final report*. Online. www.sciencewise-erc.org.uk/cms/assets/Uploads/Project-files/TrustGuide-final-Report.pdf (accessed 22 February 2017).

Lévi-Strauss, C. (1994) *The Savage Mind*. Oxford: Oxford University Press.

Locke, J. (1693) *Some Thoughts Concerning Education*. London: A. and J. Churchill.

Louv, R. (2005) *Last Child in the Woods: Saving our children from nature-deficit disorder*. Chapel Hill, NC: Algonquin Books.

MacBeath, J. (1999) *Schools Must Speak for Themselves: The case for school self-evaluation*. London: Routledge.

Martinson, J. (2011) 'Doctor, doctor, this sexist toy-selling is making me sick'. *The Guardian*, 12 December. Online. http://gu.com/p/3442f/sbl (accessed 4 July 2016).

McCahill, M. and Finn, R. (2010) 'The social impact of surveillance in three UK schools: "Angels", "devils" and "teen mums"'. *Surveillance and Society*, 7 (3), 273–89.

Mey, G. and Günther, H. (2014) *The Life Space of the Urban Child: Perspectives on Martha Muchow's classic study*. London: Transaction Publishers.

Meyer, A. (2007) 'The moral rhetoric of childhood'. *Childhood*, 14 (1), 85–104.

Morgan, N. (2016) 'Response to Education Select Committee Inquiry in PSHE'. Online. www.gov.uk/government/uploads/system/uploads/attachment_data/file/499338/Nicky_Morgan_to_Education_Select_Committee_-_10_Feb_2016--.pdf (accessed 8 July 2016).

Mortimore, P. and Sammons, P. (1997). 'Endpiece: A welcome and a riposte to critics'. In White, J. and Barber, M. (eds) *Perspectives on School Effectiveness and School Improvement*. London: Institute of Education, Bedford Way Articles.

Mortimore, P. and Whitty, G. (1997) 'Can school improvement overcome the effects of disadvantage?' Occasional paper. London: Institute of Education.

NoBullying (2015a) 'Jessica Logan: The rest of the story'. Online. http://nobullying.com/jessica-logan (accessed 8 July 2016).

— (2015b) 'The unforgettable Amanda Todd story'. Online. http://nobullying.com/amanda-todd-story/ (accessed 8 July 2016).

Nusche, D., Laveault, D., MacBeath, J., and Santiago, P. (2012) *OECD Reviews of Evaluation and Assessment in Education: New Zealand 2011*. Paris: OECD.

Odell, M. (2014) 'Should we spy on our children?'. *Daily Telegraph*, 15 November. Online. www.telegraph.co.uk/men/relationships/fatherhood/11228246/Should-we-spy-on-our-children.html (accessed 8 July 2016).

Ofcom (2011) 'Ofcom's approach to net neutrality'. 24 November. Online. http://stakeholders.ofcom.org.uk/consultations/net-neutrality/statement/ (accessed 8 July 2016).

Office for Standards in Education, Children's Services and Skills (Ofsted) (2012) 'Inspecting safeguarding'. Manchester: Ofsted. Online. http://tinyurl.com/hsugcpn (accessed 7 July 2016).

— (2013) 'School report: Prudhoe Community High School'. Manchester: Ofsted. Online. http://reports.ofsted.gov.uk/provider/files/2295845/urn/122351.pdf (accessed 5 July 2016).

— (2014) 'Inspecting E-Safety in schools: Briefing for section 5 inspection'. Manchester: Ofsted.

— (2015a) 'Safeguarding children and young people and young vulnerable adults policy'. Manchester: Ofsted. Online. www.gov.uk/government/uploads/system/uploads/attachment_data/file/446121/Safeguarding_children_and_young_people_and_young_vulnerable_adults_policy.doc (accessed 7 July 2016).

— (2015b) 'The common inspection framework: Education, skills and early years'. Manchester: Ofsted. Online. www.gov.uk/government/uploads/system/uploads/attachment_data/file/461767/The_common_inspection_framework_education_skills_and_early_years.pdf (accessed 7 July 2016).

— (2015c) 'Online safety and inspection'. Child internet safety summit, 3 July. Manchester: Ofsted. Online. www.slideshare.net/Ofstednews/childInternetsafetysummitonlinesafetyinspection (accessed 21 April 2015).

— (2016) 'School inspection handbook: Handbook for inspecting schools in England under section 5 of the Education Act 2005'. Manchester: Ofsted. Online. www.gov.uk/government/uploads/system/uploads/attachment_data/file/553942/School_inspection_handbook-section_5.pdf (accessed 16 January 2017).

Open Rights Group (2016) 'Are you being blocked?'. Online. www.blocked.org.uk (accessed 8 July 2016).

Palmer, S. (2006) *Toxic Childhood: How the modern world is damaging our children, and what we can do about it*. London: Orion.

Paoletti, J.B. (2012) *Pink and Blue: Telling the boys from the girls in America*. Bloomington: Indiana University Press.

Pardun, C., L'Engle, K., and Brown, J. (2005) 'Exposure to outcomes: Early adolescents' consumption of sexual content in six media'. *Mass Communication and Society*, 8 (2), 75–91.

Parziale, G. (2008) 'Touchless fingerprinting technology'. In Ratha, N. and Govindaraju, V. (eds) *Advances in Biometrics: Sensors, algorithms and systems*. London: Springer.

Perry, C. (2012) *An Independent Parliamentary Inquiry into Online Child Protection*. London: HMSO. Online. www.safermedia.org.uk/Images/final-report.pdf (accessed 1 November 2016).

Perry, R.W. and Quarantelli, E.L. (2005) *What is a Disaster? New answers to old questions*. New York: International Research Committee on Disasters.

Peterborough Telegraph (2016) 'Judge's warning over dangers of "sexting" following Whittlesey case'. 24 February. Online. www.peterboroughtoday.co.uk/news/crime/judge-s-warning-over-dangers-of-sexting-following-whittlesey-case-1-7229984#ixzz42ViewtZP (accessed 8 July 2016).

Phippen, A. (2009) 'Sharing personal images and videos among young people'. Exeter: South West Grid for Learning. Online. http://childnetsic.s3.amazonaws.com/downloads/Research_Highlights/UKCCIS_RH_10_Sexting.pdf (accessed 1 March 2017).

— (2010) *Online Safety Policy and Practice in the UK: An analysis of 360 Degree Safe self-review data*. Exeter: South West Grid for Learning. Online. http://swgfl.org.uk/products-services/esafety/resources/online-safety-research/Content/360analysisSept2010(2) (accessed 7 July 2016).

— (2012a) *Online Safety Policy and Practice in the UK and Internationally: An analysis of 360 Degree Safe/Generation Safe self-review data 2011*. Exeter: South West Grid for Learning. Online. http://swgfl.org.uk/news/Files/Documents/Online-Safety-Services/Online-Safety-Policy-and-Practice-in-the-UK-and-in (accessed 7 July 2016).

— (2012b) 'Sexting: An exploration of practices, attitudes and influences'. London: NSPCC. Online. www.nspcc.org.uk/globalassets/documents/research-reports/sexting-exploration-practices-attitudes-influences-report-2012.pdf (accessed 1 March 2017).

— (2013) *UK Schools Online Safety Policy and Practice Assessment 2013: Annual analysis of 360 Degree Safe self-review data*. Exeter: South West Grid for Learning. Online. http://swgfl.org.uk/products-services/esafety/resources/online-safety-research/Content/Online-Safety-Policy-and-Practice-2013 (accessed 7 July 2016).

— (2014) *UK Schools Online Safety Policy and Practice Assessment 2014: Annual analysis of 360 Degree Safe self-review data*. Exeter: South West Grid for Learning. Online. http://swgfl.org.uk/news/Files/Documents/Online-Safety-Services/360-Report-2014-Online-Safety-Policy-and-Practice (accessed 1 March 2017).

Piaget, J. and Inhelder, B. (2008) *The Psychology of the Child*. New York: Basic Books.

Pinchbeck, I. and Hewitt, M. (1969) *Children in English Society*. 2 vols. London: Routledge.

Pink News (2015) 'House of Lords votes against mandatory sex and relationship education in schools'. Online. www.pinknews.co.uk/2014/01/28/house-of-lords-votes-against-mandatory-sex-and-relationship-education-in-schools (accessed 21 April 2016).

Plant, E. and Plant, M. (1999) 'Primary prevention for young children: A comment on the UK government's 10 year drug strategy'. *International Journal of Drug Policy*, 10 (5), 385–401.

Postman, N. (1994) *The Disappearance of Childhood*. New York: Vintage.

Power, M. (1997) *The Audit Society: Rituals of verification*. Oxford: Oxford University Press.

Pring, R. (1996) 'Educating Persons: Putting education back into educational research'. *Scottish Educational Review*, 27 (2), 101–12.

Pritchard, C., Davey, J., and Williams, R. (2013) 'Who kills children? Re-examining the evidence'. *British Journal of Social Work*, 43, 1403–38.

Pugh, A.J. (2009) *Longing and Belonging: Parents, children and consumer culture*. Berkeley: University of California Press.

Quarantelli, E.L. (1998) *What is a Disaster? Perspectives on the question*. London: Routledge.

Qustodio (2016) 'How does it work? Qustodio puts full control into your hands'. Online. www.qustodio.com/en/family/how-it-works (accessed 8 July 2016).

Ringrose, J., Gill, R., Livingstone, S., and Harvey, L. (2012) 'A qualitative study of children, young people and "sexting": A report prepared for the NSPCC'. London: National Society for the Prevention of Cruelty to Children. Online. www.nspcc.org.uk/globalassets/documents/research-reports/qualitative-study-children-young-people-sexting-report.pdf (accessed 8 July 2016).

Roberts, Y. (2005) 'The one and only'. Australian *Sunday Telegraph Magazine*, 31 July.

Rousseau, J. J. (1979) *Emile, or On Education*. Trans. Bloom, A. New York: Basic Books.

Royal Society for the Prevention of Accidents (RoSPA) (2014) 'New UK figures reveal 381 drowning and other water-related deaths in 2013'. Online. www.rospa.com/media-centre/press-office/press-releases/detail/?id=1276 (accessed 5 July 2016).

— (2015) 'Taking children swimming'. Online. www.rospa.com/leisure-safety/water/advice/taking-children-swimming/ (accessed 5 July 2016).

Saluja, G., Brenner, R.A., Trumble, A.C., Smith, G.S., Schroeder, T., and Cox, C. (2006) 'Swimming pool drownings among US residents aged 5–24 years: Understanding racial/ethnic disparities.' *American Journal of Public Health*, 96 (4), 728–33.

Saracho, O. and Spodek, B. (1998) *Multiple Perspectives on Play in Early Childhood*. New York: State University of New York Press.

Schildkampa, K., Visschera, A., and Luytena, H. (2009) 'The effects of the use of a school self-evaluation instrument'. *School Effectiveness and School Improvement*, 20 (1), 69–88.

Schneier, B. (2006) 'The eternal value of privacy'. *Schneier on Security* blog. Online. www.schneier.com/essays/archives/2006/05/the_eternal_value_of.html (accessed 22 February 2017).

Schofield, R. and Midi Berry, B. (1971) 'Age at baptism in pre-industrial England'. *Population Studies*, 33, 49–63.

Scott, S., Jackson, S., and Backett-Milburn, K. (1998) 'Swings and roundabouts: Risk anxiety and the everyday worlds of children'. *Sociology*, 32 (4), 689–705.

Selwyn, N. (2011) 'It's all about standardisation: Exploring the digital (re-) configuration of school management and administration'. *Cambridge Journal of Education*, 41 (4), 473–88.

Shewbridge, C., Hulshof, M., Nusche, D., and Staehr, L.S. (2014) *OECD Reviews of Evaluation and Assessment in Education: Northern Ireland, United Kingdom*. Paris: OECD.

Shoniregun, C.A. and Crosier, S. (2008) *Securing Biometrics Applications*. London: Springer.

Siciliano, R. (2014) 'Stop! Do you really want to send that photo?'. Online. https://securingtomorrow.mcafee.com/consumer/identity-protection/love-and-tech/ (accessed 1 November 2016).

Sorokin, P. and Merton, R. (1937) 'Social time: A methodological and functional analysis'. *American Journal of Sociology*, 42 (5), 615–29.

Souter-Brown, G. (2014) *Landscape and Urban Design for Health and Wellbeing: Using healing, sensory and therapeutic gardens*. London: Routledge.

Steinberg, S.R. and Kincheloe, J.L. (2004) *Kinderculture: The corporate construction of childhood*. Boulder, CO: Westview Press.

Stoll, L. (1992) 'School self-evaluation: Another boring exercise or an opportunity for growth?'. In Riddell, S. and Brown, S. (eds) *School Effectiveness Research: Its message for school improvement*. Edinburgh: Scottish Education Department, HMSO.

Stone, N. (2011) 'The "sexting" quagmire: Criminal justice responses to adolescents' electronic transmission of indecent images in the UK and the USA'. *Youth Justice*, 11 (3), 266–81.

Strathern, M. (ed.) (2000) *Audit Cultures: Anthropological studies in accountability, ethics and the academy*. London: Routledge.

Swain, J. (2000) '"The money's good, the fame's good, the girls are good": The role of playground football in the construction of young boys' masculinity in a junior school'. *British Journal of Sociology of Education*, 21 (1), 95–109.

SWGfL (2015) 'So you got naked online'. Online. http://swgfl.org.uk/products-services/esafety/resources/So-You-Got-Naked-Online (accessed 8 July 2016).

Tandridge Trust (2015) 'Adult and child ratios'. Online. www.tandridgetrust.co.uk/index.php/swimming.html (accessed 5 July 2016).

Tang, X. (2012) 'The perverse logic of teen sexting prosecutions (and how to stop it)'. *Boston University Journal of Science and Technology Law*, 19 (1), 106.

Taylor, E. (2010) 'I spy with my little eye: Exploring the use of surveillance and CCTV in schools'. Ph.D. diss., University of Salford.

UK Government (1978) The Protection of Children Act 1978. Online. www.legislation.gov.uk/ukpga/1978/37 (accessed 8 July 2016).

— (2010) 'Academies Act 2010'. Chapter 32. Online. www.legislation.gov.uk/ukpga/2010/32/pdfs/ukpga_20100032_en.pdf (accessed 7 July 2016).

— (2011) *Prevent Strategy*. London: HMSO. Online. www.gov.uk/government/uploads/system/uploads/attachment_data/file/97976/prevent-strategy-review.pdf (accessed 8 July 2016).

— (2012) Protection of Freedoms Act 2012 c.9 Chapter 2.

— (2015a) Criminal Justice and Courts Act 2015. Online. www.legislation.gov.uk/ukpga/2015/2/contents/enacted (accessed 8 July 2016).

— (2015b) Serious Crime Act 2015. Online. www.legislation.gov.uk/ukpga/2015/9/contents/enacted/data.htm (accessed 8 July 2016).

— (2016) Online Safety Bill [HL] 2015–2016. Online. http://services.parliament.uk/bills/2015-16/onlinesafety.html (accessed 8 July 2016).

UN General Assembly (1990), 'Convention on the rights of the child', United Nations, Treaty Series, vol. 1577, 3. Online. http://treaties.un.org/doc/Publication/UNTS/Volume%201577/v1577.pdf (accessed 22 April 2016).

UNICEF (2005) *Childhood under Threat: The state of the world's children.* UNICEF: New York.

— (2016) 'FACT SHEET: A summary of the rights under the "Convention on the Rights of the Child"'. Online. www.unicef.org/crc/files/Rights_overview.pdf (accessed 8 July 2016).

Urry, J. (2003) *Global Complexity.* Cambridge: Polity.

Van der Ploeg, I. (1999) 'Written on the body: Biometrics and identity'. In Norris, C. and Wilson, D. (eds) (2006) *Surveillance, Crime and Social Control.* Aldershot: Ashgate.

Vismara, L. (2014) *A Comparison of Compensation for Personal Injury Claims in Europe.* Cologne: General Reinsurance.

Wolak, J. and Finkelhor D. (2011) 'Sexting: a typology'. Online. www.unh.edu/ccrc/pdf/CV231_Sexting%20Typology%20Bulletin_4-6-11_revised.pdf (accessed 8 July 2016).

Woods, P. (1979) *The Divided School.* London: Routledge and Kegan Paul.

Zhang, D. (2000) *Automated Biometrics: Technologies and systems.* London: Springer.

Zornado, J.L. (2001) *Inventing the Child: Culture, ideology, and the story of childhood.* New York: Garland.

Index

Index